The Vegetarian Diet *for Kidney Disease*

Preserving Kidney Function With Plant-Based Eating

Joan Brookhyser Hogan, R.D.

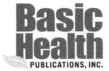

Basic Health
PUBLICATIONS, INC.

The information contained in this book is based upon the research and personal and professional experiences of the authors. It is not intended as a substitute for consulting with your physician or other healthcare provider. Any attempt to diagnose and treat an illness should be done under the direction of a healthcare professional.

The publisher does not advocate the use of any particular healthcare protocol but believes the information in this book should be available to the public. The publisher and authors are not responsible for any adverse effects or consequences resulting from the use of the suggestions, preparations, or procedures discussed in this book. Should the reader have any questions concerning the appropriateness of any procedures or preparation mentioned, the authors and the publisher strongly suggest consulting a professional healthcare advisor.

Basic Health Publications, Inc.

www.basichealthpub.com

Library of Congress Cataloging-in-Publication Data

Hogan, Joan B.
  The vegetarian diet for kidney disease : preserving kidney function with plant-based eating / Joan B. Hogan.
      p. cm.
  Includes bibliographical references and index.
  ISBN 978-1-59120-266-0 Paperback
  ISBN 978-1-68162-670-3 Hardback

  1. Kidneys—Diseases—Diet therapy. 2. Vegetarianism. 3. Vegetarian cookery. I. Title.
  RC903.H64   2009
  616.6'10654—dc22

                                              2009044165

Editor: Roberta W. Waddell
Typesetting/Book design: Gary A. Rosenberg
Cover design: Mike Stromberg

Printed in the United States of America

10   9   8   7   6   5   4   3   2

Contents

To My Mother,
who instilled in me the importance of nutrition
in combating disease and promoting health

Acknowledgments

I wish to express my thanks to the following people who were instrumental in the development and publication of this book.

Carol Kinzner, R.N., A.R.N.P., Kathy Harvey, M.S., R.D., Kerri Wiggins, M.S., R.D., Maude Valentine, R.N., Anne Mesaros, R.D., C.D.E.; Judy Clark, Patti Shepard, and Amy Putnum.

In this second edition, I want to thank nephrologist Dr. Paul Schneider, Joni Pagenkemper, and Kathy Harvey. I also want to acknowledge Joy Pierson and Bart Potenza for giving me permission to adapt their wonderful vegetarian recipes from *The Candle Café Cookbook* for this edition. And my thanks go as well to my publisher Norman Goldfind. I very much appreciate him giving me the opportunity to republish my work in a way that reaches the many who need it.

In addition, I want to thank the many patients I have worked with over the years who have given me the motivation to write this book. And finally I want to thank my husband and best friend, Pat Hogan, who provided ongoing encouragement and support for my dreams: to have this book published and to make a difference in the lives of those people who are coping with chronic kidney disease.

Introduction

PLANT PROTEIN FOR HEALTH AND DISEASE

When I first became a dietitian over thirty years ago, vegetarianism and chronic kidney disease did not mix. If you were a vegetarian, you were advised to let go of your herbivore ways. If you were curious about becoming a vegetarian, you were discouraged. The research at that time saw plant proteins as inferior to animal proteins. This inferiority was thought to cause people with chronic kidney disease to become sicker or more uremic from their condition. In addition, it was thought that plant proteins were too high in many of the minerals that needed to be restricted in chronic kidney disease, thus causing more complications.

In the last fifteen years, however, further research has changed this viewpoint, which is now known not to be the case. Vegan, lacto-ovo vegetarian, or occasional vegetarian eating *can* fit with chronic kidney disease. And vegetarianism is not only acceptable, it is being found superior to meat-based diets in the prevention and treatment of chronic kidney disease. By following the guidelines in this book you can begin, or continue, a plant-based diet to help, not harm, your kidney health.

WHAT IF YOU ARE NOT A VEGETARIAN

If you are not a vegetarian, you can still find value in this book. Even eating a partial vegetarian diet, or alternating between a vegetarian and non-vegetarian diet, can be of value in chronic kidney-disease treatment. This book will give you guidelines to working with meat, fish, or poultry, if you so choose, while helping you maintain a healthy, safe diet for your level of kidney function.

The information provided is not only intended to promote a healthy plant-based diet, but to help you in planning the healthiest diet possible for long-term health and fitness. In the years I've worked with people who have kidney disease, I have seen some die, not from their kidney disease, but from other conditions, such as cancer, complications of diabetes, heart disease, or infections. A well-planned diet is at the forefront of this battle of health before you and will help reduce your risk of complications—such a diet is not only necessary for plant-based eating, but also for healthy eating in general.

WORKING WITH YOUR HEALTHCARE PROFESSIONALS

This book is not meant to replace your medical care. In addition to good nutritional management, treatment for chronic kidney disease works best by making routine visits to your physician and following his or her recommendations for the medical aspects of your treatment.

This book has been designed to help those with a glomerular filtration rate (GFR) greater than 30 cc/minute who are not receiving dialysis

A Note about the Overall Focus of this Book

There are many books, journal articles, Internet writings, etc., concerned with the origins of chronic kidney disease (CKD). Although reasons for this disease are scattered throughout the book, it does not focus on them. Instead, it begins with the assumption that the reader either has chronic kidney disease, or knows someone who does, and is using this book as a practical how-to handbook for optimum treatment and therapy.

treatment, or those with a glomerular filtration rate less than 15 ml/minute who are receiving dialysis treatment. If you are experiencing kidney disease with a creatinine clearance less than 30ml/minute, I strongly recommend that you augment the information in this book with professional assistance. In addition to being closely monitored by a physician who specializes in kidney disease, this would include seeking the individualized counseling of a dietitian who is certified in the specialty of renal (kidney) nutrition. Such dietitians can be found by contacting:

The National Kidney Foundation at 1-800-622-9010

The American Dietetic Association at 1-800-877-1600

TERMINOLOGY

Even though I have attempted to minimize unnecessary medical jargon, many such words are needed to help in the understanding and self-treatment of your disease. The Glossary and Appendix A will assist you in understanding the terminology and laboratory tests used in this book.

A NOTE TO THE PROFESSIONAL

This book is not meant to replace professional nutritional management or healthcare. However, I often find patients who desire to self-treat or seek resources outside the traditional healthcare arena and, as a result, receive dangerous or harmful advice. Since my first edition of this book, I have found this to be true on several occasions and have been pleased that this publication was available to provide accurate guidance. Many of these people were able to share this information with their healthcare professional, thereby facilitating better treatment care. Since the National Kidney Foundation's Kidney Disease Outcomes Quality Initiative (K/DOQI) identified the stages of chronic kidney disease, an awareness and treatment of chronic kidney disease has been initiated earlier. Nutritional management, predominantly in plant-based diets, is part of that early intervention. I have attempted to address vegetarianism in a way that facilitates a dialogue between you and your patients who read this. I feel that educated patients can have the best outcome. With increased the use of the Internet, people can be at risk for inaccurate resources. In an effort to combat possible misinformation, I have made valid, safe information available to those who seek it. As a healthcare professional, it is my hope that you can utilize this book in the care of your patients who desire a vegetarian lifestyle.

1

The Benefits of Vegetarianism

THE VEGETARIAN LIFESTYLE

The benefits of vegetarianism in chronic kidney disease begin with prevention of the disease itself. Vegetarianism is one of many lifestyle components that can help prevent complications that lead to a decline in kidney function. High blood pressure places more pressure on the kidney's vascular system and can cause damage to the kidney. High lipid levels in the blood can lead to blood-vessel narrowing, heart disease, and kidney problems. Plant-based eating is low in fat and high in the nutrients that can prevent these diseases or delay their complications, leading the way to preserving the health of your kidneys.

If you have just found out you have kidney disease, a plant-based diet can slow down its progression and possibly help other problems associated with that disease. Research suggests the amino acids that make up plant-based proteins may be less stressful on the kidneys than animal-based proteins and, in turn, may slow down the progression of kidney damage. This slowing of the damage happens by decreasing pressure on the glomeruli, or filters, of the kidney, which can help control blood pressure and decreased proteinuria (protein in the urine).

Protein loss in the urine is a sign of progressive kidney damage. The more protein loss, the more kidney damage. If you have diabetes, a properly planned vegetarian diet with consistent carbohydrates will help control your diabetes, and this improved control also lessens the progression of kidney loss.

If you have chronic kidney disease and require dialysis, a vegetarian diet can also be of benefit to you. Cardiac disease is the number-one reason for death in people on dialysis, and by helping to decrease harmful fats or lipids in the blood, a vegetarian diet can decrease this health risk. In addition, a plant-based diet may lower homocysteine levels in the blood. Homocysteine levels, a marker of heart disease, are often higher in kidney disease.

Plants, not animals, are the source of phytochemicals. The benefits and functions of phytochemicals—also known as allyl sulfides, ellagic acid, indoles, isoflavones, phenolic acids, reservatol, and saponins—continue to show promise in many chronic illnesses. It is now known that these plant chemicals are potent antioxidants, and kidney diseases, such as glomerulernephritis, may greatly benefit from a diet high in antioxidants. In addition, as it is for people without kidney disease, a strong immune system is very important for those with kidney disease. A diet high in these nutrients can help your immune system remain strong, preventing other diseases, infections, or possible cancers.

Fiber is most abundant in plant-based diets. A high-fiber diet plays a role in disease management and prevention. Your chronic kidney disease may require many medications that can be constipating, but insoluble fiber may help relieve the constipating effect of these medications. Soluble fiber can help with diabetes and cholesterol management. Foods high in fiber are also high in prebiotics and probiotics, which further assist the body's defense mechanism. In planning a diet that is plentiful in plants and minimal in processed foods and animal proteins, you are in the best position to obtain adequate fiber overall.

In the following chapters, these topics will be addressed in more detail to help you plan a safe, healthy, and tasty diet for the management of your chronic kidney disease.

MYTHS OF VEGETARIANISM IN KIDNEY DISEASE

There are many myths that surround vegetarianism in kidney disease. These myths are based on the assumption that plant proteins are incomplete, unbalanced, or even dangerous in kidney disease. This is no truer of a plant-based diet than it is of one that is animal-based. The three myths that follow are the most common you will hear.

Myth 1—Vegetarian Diets Do Not Provide Quality Protein

Quality protein no longer equals animal protein. Historically, animal proteins were thought to be the only good-quality protein that provided all of your amino acids in perfect balance without the concern of excess nitrogen wastes.

Early in the twentieth century, protein quality was assessed on the basis of how a particular protein supported the growth of rapidly developing baby rats. This technique was called protein efficiency ratio (PER). These studies indicated that eggs and other animal products had a higher biological value of protein than plant products, or, in other words, they made healthier rats. As a result, this led to the assumption that humans also needed these same proteins. This theory is now history, for we are not rats. The growth, and therefore the protein needs, of rats are different from that of humans.

In 1989, the International Food and Agriculture Organization (FAO), the World Health Organization (WHO), and the United States Department of Agriculture (USDA) adopted the Protein Digestibility-Corrected Amino Acid Score (PDCAAS) as the official assay for the evaluation of protein quality. The PDCAAS takes into account a protein's essential amino-acid composition, corrected for digestibility and referenced to the two- to five-year-old human-requirement pattern. This new method of evaluating protein quality found that some plant proteins provide high-quality protein as well.

Several studies have looked at the impact of animal and plant protein on the function of healthy kidneys. Overall, studies show that when people eat animal-protein diets, their kidneys have to work harder to filter the blood and remove wastes than they do with plant-protein diets. The reason for this is not clear, but it is thought that the cause may be the differences between the amino-acid makeup of the two protein sources; the amino-acid combinations in animal protein are more difficult for the kidneys to filter than the amino-acid combinations in plant protein.

There are only a few cautions to eating a high-quality plant protein. The amino acids may be unbalanced, and if you were to eat only grains (i.e., gluten, millet, pasta, rice, seitan) for your protein, this could result in some deficiencies. Therefore, in order to maximize your amino-acid profile, eating a variety of plant proteins is recommended. This includes such foods as dried cooked beans and legumes, soy products, and a variety of quality protein grains. (See Chapter 6 for additional information.)

Myth 2—Vegetarian Diets Cannot Provide You with Enough Protein

Over 50 percent of the world population meets their protein needs by grains alone. Additionally, 65 percent of the world population meets their protein needs by plant proteins alone. Plant proteins *can* meet all your protein requirements. Plant proteins can provide a quality diet when a low-protein diet is required. Plant proteins can provide a quality high-protein diet if you require dialysis treatment. The only time you may need additional help to make sure you are getting enough nutritional balance from your vegetarian diet is if your GFR is below 30 ml/minute and you are not on renal replacement therapy (RRT), such as dialysis. In this case, you may require the help of a registered dietitian who specializes in kidney disease to plan a diet that adequately meets your nutritional needs.

Myth 3—Vegetarian Diets Are Too High in Phosphorus and Potassium to be Used in Kidney Disease

It is estimated that 100 percent of the phosphorus from processed foods is absorbed, and 70 percent of the phosphorus from animal products is absorbed, but only 50 percent of the phosphorus from plant foods is absorbed. So even though some plant proteins are higher in phosphorus, this higher phosphorus content is not as well absorbed as it is from animal and processed-food sources. This is because many plant proteins have high levels of phytates, substances that act to block the absorption of phosphorus.

In certain plant proteins, such as beans and nuts, potassium can be quite concentrated, but these foods have other nutrients that can be of benefit to your health. With careful planning, most of these beneficial foods can be worked into your diet, and modifying portion sizes may be all you need to do.

2

The Stages
of Kidney Disease

TYPES OF KIDNEY FAILURE

There are two classifications of kidney failure, acute and chronic. Acute kidney failure happens very rapidly. You are often hospitalized and treated, and you usually regain kidney function. Diet changes needed for acute kidney failure are usually temporary and may be required in the acute phase only, although a continued vegetarian lifestyle can help you maintain your health and immunity to prevent further kidney damage. This is because the vegetarian diet is low in sodium and is optimal for health and disease prevention.

This book is written to address the needs of the second type of kidney failure—chronic kidney disease—a progressive type of kidney failure that does not usually improve. With proper medical treatment, however, chronic kidney disease can be slowed down or kept from progressing. Nutrition is a key component of that care.

KNOWING YOUR NUMBERS

One of the most important numbers you will need to become familiar with in managing your diet and kidney-disease progression is your glomerular filtration rate (GFR). This gives you the best measurement of your kidney function and will make you more aware of your nutritional and medical needs.

The most accurate way to determine your GFR is by measuring a twenty-four-hour collection of urine. However, since this can be very cumbersome, other, easier methods of calculating these numbers are frequently used now. Some laboratories will use an easier formula that can be part of your routine blood chemistries. Or you can calculate a number, known as a creatinine clearance, on your own, following the Cockcroft-Gault Formula below. All you will need is your creatinine from your current blood chemistries.

If you are a female:

Creatinine Clearance = 140 minus age multiplied by ideal weight in kilograms divided by the creatinine × 72, then multiplied by .85

or

$$\text{Creatinine Clearance} = \frac{(140 - \text{age}) \times \text{ideal weight in kilograms}}{\text{creatinine} \times 72} \times .85$$

Calculating your creatinine clearance will give you a close approximation of your GFR or the filtering ability of your kidneys.

According to the National Kidney Foundation, the stages of kidney disease can be classified as shown in Table 2.1. By looking on the table for your own GFR or creatinine clearance you can determine what stage

Diet and Supplements
Maintain Consistent GFR

Seventy-five-year-old Robert came to see me for Stage 3 kidney disease, cause unknown. He was used to eating a diet high in animal proteins. I instructed him to increase his soy-based protein and limit his intake of high-sodium foods. I also told him to use the natural anti-inflammatory agents, omega-3 fatty acids and glucosamine, to help with his arthritis. Robert took my advice, and five years later, he continued to maintain a GFR that was consistent with Stage 3 kidney disease.

of chronic kidney disease you have. Please note: These descriptions and diet guidelines are general and may vary depending on your type of kidney disease, other medical problems you are experiencing, or the medications you are taking.

TABLE 2.1. STAGES OF KIDNEY DISEASE		
STAGE	GFR	DESCRIPTION
1	90 cc/min	Kidney damage, protein in the urine, normal filtration
2	60–89cc/min	Kidney damage with a mild decrease in filtration kidney
3	30–59 cc/min	Moderate decrease in filtration
4	15–29 cc/min	Severe decline in filtration
5	< 15 cc/min	Kidney failure—dialysis or transplant will be needed soon

END-STAGE RENAL DISEASE

Although many people continue to function well with a GFR below 15, you may no longer be able sustain your health without renal replacement therapy, where your choices are dialysis treatment or a kidney transplant. Your doctor may start to talk to you about these options. If you are not on dialysis, your diet may need more restrictions. If you are on dialysis, your diet needs become even more specific because your kidneys are no longer able to filter nutrients effectively. The following chapters will help guide you concerning which nutrients you should be eating, and in what quantities, depending on your stage and type of kidney disease.

3

Common Problems Associated with Chronic Kidney Disease

Many side effects of kidney disease can occur. Some of these problems are not necessarily due to kidney disease but to other diseases, such as cancer, diabetes, or heart disease, that occur with kidney disease. Following are some of the more common problems and the suggested nutritional treatments for them.

THIRST

Feeling thirsty is a very common problem with kidney disease. The cause can be due to urea, a solute (waste product) building up in your blood. Urea is giving your body a signal to dilute it. In addition, it can be due to a high-salt diet, some medications, or if you have diabetes, it can be caused by high blood sugars. Being extra thirsty can be a problem if you are receiving dialysis, not urinating regularly, or have edema (water retention in the tissues). If you are on dialysis and you drink too much liquid, it stays with you until your next dialysis treatment. If you are taking water pills and you take in excess liquid, the pills do not work as well. In either case, excess fluid can put pressure on your heart, causing congestive heart failure.

Ways to Treat Thirst

- If you are dialyzing, make sure that you receive your full treatment time. If you are constantly late for your treatment or come off early, you may be missing vital minutes to *clean* your blood more thoroughly. This means there will be higher levels of urea that will trigger thirst. This thirst may cause you to drink more than can be removed during your treatment.

- If you have diabetes, watch your blood sugars. If needed, see your diabetes specialist or a diabetes educator to re-adjust your insulin or oral medication for better control. With kidney failure, insulin often needs changing.

- Check the salt in your diet. Overall, a vegetarian diet is low in sodium, but if you are using a lot of meat substitutes, you may be getting more than your recommended sodium allowance for the day. If you are using a meat replacement that has more than 700 mg of sodium per serving you may want to find another product. (See Appendix D for product-information sheets on some of these foods.)

- Limit your fluid intake to $1-1^{1}/_{2}$ quarts per day.

- Review your medications with a qualified pharmacist. The pharmacist can tell you which medications are making you thirsty. One example is Benedryl or other antihistamines. Discuss the medication with your physician to see if you can be switched to other brands, or maybe discontinue them altogether.

TASTE

Many people with kidney disease complain of changes in taste for foods. This is particularly true when your kidney function is down to about 25–30 percent. This is due to a urea buildup in your blood and often improves with regular dialysis. However, this change in taste can also be caused by a zinc deficiency. If you have been eating poorly, you may not be receiving enough zinc and may require supplementation. Ask a nutritionally aware physician to test your zinc level. Do not supplement your diet with additional zinc until you find out what your level is because supplementing with zinc when you are not deficient can cause other nutrient imbalances in your body.

NAUSEA OR VOMITING

It is not uncommon to have bouts of nausea or even vomiting with kidney disease. This is most common right before you start dialysis or when your GFR is less than 20 ml/min. If you are experiencing this problem, you may need to supplement your diet with a high-calorie protein drink. There are several on the market, and which one you pick will depend on your medical problems.

- Ensure Plus and Resource Plus. These are moderately high-calorie and high-protein drinks and need to be used cautiously if your potassium or phosphorus levels are high.

- Glucerna or Resource Diabetic. These are moderately high-calorie and high-protein drinks, low in carbohydrates and high in fiber. Often used by people with diabetes for better blood-sugar control. They need to be used cautiously if your potassium or phosphorus is high.

- Suplena. Often used to provide a lot of calories when you have very little kidney function, but are not receiving dialysis. It is very low in protein.

- NV Renal or Nepro. These very high calorie protein drinks are given when receiving dialysis. Somewhat more expensive than Ensure or Resource, they are often recommended when calories and protein are needed without a lot of potassium and phosphorus.

These products may have to be special ordered by your pharmacy, or you can contact the company yourself. See Resources in back for contact numbers.

If you are experiencing ongoing problems with nausea, it may help to follow the suggestions for people with diabetes in Chapter 4.

CONSTIPATION

Some of the medications you take for your kidney disease may cause constipation. This can be very frustrating. Making sure to eat high fiber foods can help a great deal. Choose fruits and vegetables with skins. Select whole grains, such as barley, brown rice, and whole wheat bread, and add in a high-fiber cereal, too. See the following list for further suggestions. If you are not used to high fiber cereals, it is always a good idea to add them to your diet gradually. If you do not do this, you could experience additional stomach and digestion discomfort.

Fiber supplements, such as Unifiber, Benefiber, or psyllium capsules, can also help constipation. They are tasteless and can easily be added to your food. Information on how to buy these supplements can be found in Resources in back.

TABLE 3.1.   GOOD SOURCES OF FIBER

FOOD SOURCE (IN HALF-CUP SERVINGS WHERE NOT SPECIFIED)	AVERAGE GRAMS OF FIBER
Cooked whole grains, such as barley, brown rice, bulgar, or couscous	3–6
Dried cooked beans, such as black, garbonzo, or pinto beans	5–7
Fresh apples with skin	3–4
Fresh blackberries, raspberries, or strawberries	2–4
Fresh pears most types	3–4
Kellogg's All Bran, ready to eat	9
Meatless ground meat	3–4
Oatmeal, cooked, regular—non-instant	4
Popcorn, 3 cups	3–4
Raw vegetables with skin	2–4
Veggieburgers, most brands—1 patty	3–4
Wheatena, cooked	6
Wholegrain pasta	2–4

DIARRHEA

There can be several reasons for diarrhea with kidney disease. Most often it is due to medications or infections. If you have diabetes, this can also be the cause of this problem. Some of the following ideas may help you, but if the problem persists even after trying these things, make sure to discuss this with your physician. Prolonged diarrhea can lead to poor absorption of nutrients, which will further compromise your health.

- Milk products can sometimes cause diarrhea. They are high in a sugar called lactose that some people do not tolerate well. If you think you are lactose intolerant, try eliminating all milk, cheese, pudding, yogurt, or foods made with dry milk powder for a while and see if this helps your symptoms.

- Sometimes the use of sugar-substitute products, such as sugar-free beverages, candy, cookies, or puddings, can cause stomach upset and diarrhea. These foods contains sugar alcohol, such as mannitol, sorbitol, or xylitol, that can be difficult for some people to digest.

- The following foods will help with diarrhea by absorbing water and slowing down digestion, at the same time providing bulk and form to your stool.
  - Apple or pear with skin, 1 small
  - Applesauce, $1/2$ cup
  - Cornflakes, 1 cup
  - Corn (fresh or canned), $1/2$ cup
  - Fresh salads (carrots, cucumbers, green pepper, lettuce), 1 cup
  - Oatmeal or grits, $3/4$ cup
  - Pasta, $3/4$ cup
  - White rice, $3/4$ cup

- Try congee: $1/2$ cup rice cooked in 2–3 cups of water—eat small amounts throughout the day.

• An amino acid called L-glutamine has shown promising relief for diarrhea problems. L-glutamine supplements can be purchased at your
health food store. A dose of 500 mg two times per day is recommended. Contacts for buying this supplement are in Resources in
back.

• If you have been on a course of antibiotics followed by diarrhea, probiotics such as S. cerevisiae or S. boulardii may be of help.

ITCHING

Itching is very common in kidney disease and can worsen as your kidney function decreases. There are several reasons for this, including high
toxin levels, too much phosphorus in your blood, or a deficiency in
omega-3 fatty acids. Try the following if you itch.

• Have your phosphorus level checked. If it is high, make sure you are
limiting your milk group to the amount allowed. Check the types of
beans you are using to make sure they are the lower phosphorus ones.
If you are taking binders, make sure you do not forget to take them.
Always take them right before you eat to get the greatest benefit. (See
Phosphorus, Chapter 5.)

• If you have uremia and are on dialysis, make sure you are getting
your full dialysis treatment time. Even missing five minutes can result
in inadequate urea being removed. High blood-urea levels can cause
itching.

• Add at least 1 gram of omega-3 fatty acids to your daily diet.

• Health food stores carry high-quality, non-allergenic, fragrance-free
lotions that can help with itching skin.

POOR HEALING

With kidney disease you may find you do not heal quickly. Good nutrition is going to be your best catalyst to heal. If you are not healing well
after surgery, or from other injuries or trauma, try the following.

- Review your diet. Are you eating all your food groups?

- Weigh yourself. Are you losing weight? If so, talk with a nutritionally aware doctor or go to a dietitian to learn ways to increase your calories. Or add more fat calories to your diet. Again, make sure you are eating all the servings in your food groups.

- Take a renal-approved vitamin supplement.

- Take a 15-mg supplement of zinc per day.

- Take 300 mg of vitamin C two times per day. However, limit this to only a few months—long-term high-vitamin-C intake can be dangerous to people with kidney disease.

- If you are still having troubles healing, ask your doctor to prescribe a vitamin A ointment. This will often help with healing. *Do not take vitamin A supplements,* only topical vitamin A is recommended.

- Try arginine. This is an amino acid that helps with wound healing. You can get arginine from the health food store. Take twice a day for the best results. If the supplement is going to work, you will see results in two weeks. (See Resources in back for information about this supplement.)

- If you have diabetes, make sure your blood sugar stays below 200 mg/dl for good healing.

Restless Legs

Unusual leg twitching can often occur with kidney disease. This is a frustrating problem that can normally be resolved by exercising and taking magnesium. Some of this problem may be due to your kidney disease alone, but certain nutrients, such as excess caffeine or alcohol, can also impact the problem. In addition, deficiencies of biotin, carnitine, or iron can be factors. Ask to have your carnitine level checked to see if you are deficient. A supplement of L-carnitine, 500 mg per day, may help if you are deficient. Make sure your renal vitamin has biotin added. If not, find one that does.

If you are iron-deficient, make sure you are being checked and treated. Low ferritin levels are common in kidney disease, so it is most important to have your physician check your ferritin level, which measures iron storage, as this is often low in restless legs. Even with a normal hematocrit, hemoglobin, or serum iron level, a ferritin level between 50 and 100 mg/dl is recommended with this disorder. If your ferritin is less than this, taking oral iron, at least 300 mg per day, up to three times per day, is recommended. Good iron supplements for low ferritins are polysaccharide iron complexes, such as Niferex or Proferrin, an iron polypeptide.

Other nutrients worth checking for are B_{12}, folic acid, and, importantly, magnesium, because a deficiency of these can contribute to this disorder. If all these blood tests are normal, medications called dopamine agonists can help resolve your symptoms. Discuss this with your physician.

SEXUAL DYSFUNCTION

This problem can be uncomfortable to discuss, but sexuality can have a huge impact on your quality of life. There are many factors that effect sexuality and kidney disease. Most are not directly related to nutrition, but can be affected by your nutritional choices.

Anemia, diabetes, high blood pressure, untreated high phosphorus levels, vascular disease, and waste-product buildup can impact sexual function, sexual comfort, and sexual desire. Medications often required with kidney disease can further effect sexual complications.

- If you have diabetes, good blood-sugar control will help prevent circulation problems to genital organs.

- Low energy levels can contribute to sexual dysfunction, so managing anemia is important to maintaining your energy level. You can do this by having your B_{12}, iron, and folate levels tested, and by taking additional amounts of these supplements, if indicated.

- Healthy serum lipids can help limit the progression of heart disease.

Your plant-based diet will naturally help with lipid management, but you may also want to look at the information in Chapter 5.

- Sodium and weight control will help with your blood pressure and improve circulation to the genital organs.

- Waste-product buildup can be overcome by keeping within the protein limits set by your healthcare provider. If you are receiving dialysis treatment, it will be important to receive your whole treatment time. Keeping your body free of waste will help it function better.

- Taking the supplement package noted in Table 7.1 will ensure that you are receiving the right micronutrients.

Other Supplements

Several additional supplements are suggested as remedies for sexual function. Some, such as yohimbe, are dangerous, but there are others with potential benefits that are worth mentioning. The following are supplements that show the most promise without risk to your kidney function.

Note: As with all supplements, make sure your healthcare providers know you are taking these products.

Alpha Lipoic Acid is a fatty acid and strong antioxidant that is manufactured in the body. Supplemental doses can help with neuropathy and loss of sensation, particularly in diabetes, but it can also help people who do not have diabetes. A recommended dose of 600 mg per day is suggested.

L–Carnitine can be helpful in sexual dysfunction, according to a few isolated studies. Increasing your oral supplement of carnitine to 2 g per day may be of benefit. (See Chapter 7 for information on this nutrient as part of a maintenance package.)

Omega-3 fatty acids are not only good for your overall health, they can be helpful for sexual function as well. Increasing your maintenance dosage by 2 grams a day may further benefit you. As anti-inflammatory agents, omega-3 fatty acids have a therapeutic application in anemia, heart disease, high triglycerides, and pruritis (itching), all of which can indirectly affect sexual desire and performance. (See Chapter 7 for information on this supplement as part of a maintenance package.)

Probiotic supplementation may be helpful for women. Often the vaginal flora can be disrupted by antibiotics and disease complications, and probiotics help normalize vaginal flora. The probiotics lactobacillus rhamnosus and lactobacillus reuteri are the best cultures for this.

Saw palmetto is an herb used for treating benign prostrate hypertrophy, prostate-cancer prevention, and possibly erectile dysfunction. A usual dose is 160–320 mg per day.

Do not forget overall good nutrition. If you are losing weight or are tired, consider individual diet counseling with a registered dietitian to make sure you are meeting all your nutritional needs.

WHEN TO SEEK PROFESSIONAL HELP

This book is intended to help you plan your diet, but there may be times when you will require the help of a registered dietitian who specializes in kidney disease and is supportive of your desire to eat vegetarian.

Some signs that you may require more help in planning your diet include the following:

- You lose more that 10 percent of your body weight in three months;

- You have very high potassium and/or phosphorus levels, which you are unable to get into the normal range on your own;

- Your kidney function is below 20 percent;

- Your albumin, a protein in your blood, is less than 3.r mg/dl (ask your doctor to check your level);

- You are nauseated and are having trouble finding things you can eat.

4

Kidney Disease and Other Diseases

DIABETES AND KIDNEY DISEASE

More than 50 percent of kidney disease is due to diabetes. If you have both diabetes and kidney disease, you can feel a little overwhelmed. You may wonder what, if anything, there is to eat, but actually the diabetes and kidney diets can be easily combined. One of the best ways to delay the progression of kidney disease is to control your blood sugar. Blood-sugar monitoring is recommended for anyone with diabetes, whether on oral medications, insulin, or diet alone. Maintaining good blood-sugar control is the best way to avoid complications related to diabetes and kidney disease.

Keep Track of Your Blood Sugar

If you are on dialysis, or if you are in Stage 4 or 5, you may begin to notice changes in how much insulin you require. This is because your kidney is no longer able to process and eliminate insulin, and as a result it stays in your body longer. Keeping track of changes in your blood sugar and your insulin reactions will help you and your doctor make the best adjustments in your insulin dosage.

Keep Meals Regular

No matter what your schedule is, a regular routine is best. For times when you are tired or busy, keep easy-to-fix foods on hand. If you are sick or nauseous, you still need to eat because this will keep your blood

Improved Regime, Improved Results

Duncan M., a fifty-year-old gentleman, came to see me for progressive kidney failure, Stage 3, due to Type II diabetes. For many years, he had been eating many processed foods and an excess of animal protein. I started him on a plant-based diet, and got him to stop eating processed foods that were high in sodium. Duncan also began to exercise regularly, and after only three months of this improved regime, his GFR level increased to Stage 2.

sugar stable. Also, be sure the drinks or food you keep on hand are easy to digest.

Keep Your Carbohydrates Consistent

It is very important to your long-term health to make sure the amount of insulin you take is appropriate for the amount of carbohydrates you eat, and also make sure that the amounts of these foods are consistent from meal to meal. This will help stabilize your blood sugar. Table 4.1 below lists the grams of carbohydrates in frequently eaten foods.

Diet Reverses GFR

Andrew was a thirty-year-old man with Type I diabetes who came to see me as a referral from his doctor after his GFR had placed him at Stage 4 kidney disease (he had previously been Stage 1). He'd been following a high-protein diet, twice what had been recommended for him, and a very low-carbohydrate diet intended for weight loss and blood-sugar control. After explaining the risks of a high animal-protein diet, and educating him about limiting the excessive amounts of refined carbohydrates he had been ingesting (mainly in the rice he had been eating), Andrew followed my advice and was able to control his blood-sugar levels and lose weight safely. Further, these steps allowed his GFR to return to a level consistent with Stage 1 kidney disease.

TABLE 4.1. CARBOHYDRATE SOURCES		
FOOD GROUP	SERVINGS	CARBOHYDRATES (GRAMS)
Bread	1 slice	15
Fruits	1 piece	15
Grains, rice, pasta, cereal (cooked)	1/2 cup	15
Milk	8 oz	12
Vegetables	1/2 cup cooked, 1 cup raw	5

KEEP EASY-TO-PREPARE FOODS FOR NAUSEA

The following is a list of foods that are easily tolerated by most people when they are sick. Each food will provide 15 grams of carbohydrates in the serving size listed. To get 150–200 grams of carbohydrates for one day, choose at least ten of the foods below. It is a good idea to have some of these foods on hand in case you get sick.

Bread and Starches

1 slice bread
1/2 cup hot cereal
6 crackers (Ritz, Hi Ho, or saltines)
3 graham crackers (2 1/2 inch square)
6 vanilla wafers
1 small baked potato
1/2 cup mashed potatoes
1 oz (1/4 cup) unsalted pretzels
1/3 cup rice

Milk or Milk-Substitute Products

1/4 cup milkshake
1 1/2 cups tofu milkshake (see Recipes in Chapter 8)
1/4 cup pudding, regular
1/2 cup pudding, low-calorie
1/2 cup ice cream
1/2 cup eggnog, commercial
1 cup milk
1 1/2 cups soy milk
1 cup plain yogurt or artificially sweetened yogurt

Fruit Juices and Other Sweets

$1/2$ cup fruit juice

$1/2$ cup unsweetened applesauce

$1/2$ cup regular soft drink

$1/2$ twin popsicle

1 tablespoon regular jams or jellies

1 tablespoon white or granular sugar

1 tablespoon honey

$1/4$ cup sherbet

1 cup cream soup

$1/2$ cup regular gelatin

$1/2$ can Resource or Ensure Diabetic

Sample Menu for Carbohydrate Replacement When You Are Sick or Nauseous

	Meal	Carbohydrates
First meal	$1/2$ cup hot cereal	15 grams
	1 cup milk or $1^1/_2$ cups soy milk	15 grams
	1 tablespoon sugar	15 grams
Second meal	4 oz 7-Up	15 grams
Third meal	$1/2$ cup apple juice	15 grams
	8 animal crackers	15 grams
Fourth meal	1 cup cream soup	15 grams
Fifth meal	$1/4$ cup pudding	15 grams
Sixth meal	$1/2$ cup 7-Up	15 grams
	1 piece dry toast	15 grams
TOTAL		150 grams

Know What to Do if Your Blood Sugar Drops Low

Test your blood sugar frequently. If your blood sugar goes low, use sugar in water, or regular pop or soda, to raise it. *Do not* use juice if you can avoid it. Juice is high in potassium and may cause your potassium to go too high.

A blood sugar less than 70 mg/dl is considered a low blood sugar. This should be treated with readily available sugar, such as 3–5 Life-Savers or $1/_2$ cup regular soda.

A blood sugar greater than 300 mg/dl is considered a high blood sugar. If this occurs, and you are not ill, try a little activity and recheck your blood sugar in four hours. If it is still greater than 300 mg/dl after four hours, you should contact your physician.

Know how to take your diabetes medications.

It is important to know the right time to take your diabetes medications as this can impact the effectiveness of the medication and the control of your blood sugars. Check with your doctor, pharmacist, or dietitian if you are unsure.

HEART DISEASE AND HIGH BLOOD PRESSURE IN KIDNEY DISEASE

Sometimes it's hard to tell which came first, the kidney disease or the heart disease. Regardless, kidney disease can often be linked to circulatory and vascular heart disease. In addition, high cholesterol levels are a consistent feature of certain types of kidney disease and may be an important risk factor for progressive hardening of the arteries and progression of kidney damage. According to the DASH (Dietary Approaches to Stop Hypertension) diet, plant-based eating can lower your risk of heart disease and high blood pressure. Plant-based diets are higher in fiber and lower in total fat, saturated fat, and cholesterol than non-vegetarian diets, and vegetarians in general have lower rates of heart disease and hypertension.

Lipid Profile

An important step in the prevention of heart disease is to know your

lipid profile and the different *types* of fat in your blood. If you have not
done so, have your blood lipid panel checked. Based on recommendations from the American Heart Association, Table 4.2 will help you determine what your results mean. Your lipid panel helps to determine your
own personal risk for heart disease and stroke.

TABLE 4.2. WHAT IS YOUR LIPID PANEL			
TYPE OF FAT	ACCEPTABLE	BORDERLINE	HIGH-RISK
Total cholesterol	Below 200	200–239	Greater than 240
HDL (high-density lipoproteins)	Greater than 60	35–45	Less than 40 for men; 50 for women
LDL (low-density lipoproteins)	Less than 100	100–130	Greater than 160
Triglycerides	Less than 150	150–199	Greater than 200

Once you know your own lipid profile, you can begin to eat in a
way to make your lipid profile as healthy as possible. Each type of fat
you eat affects your lipids differently. (See Table 5.6 in Chapter 5 for
more information on fats.)

In addition, continue to follow a vegetarian diet and make use of
these tips.

• Choose low-fat milk or milk-substitute products.

• Choose high-fiber foods, such as *fresh* fruits and vegetables (not
canned). Use wholegrain breads instead of processed or white bread
or grain products. A fiber intake of 25–30 g per day is recommended.
(See Fiber section in Chapter 3.)

• Watch your labels and serving sizes. Even foods that say *trans-fatty-
acid-free* or *fat-free* are not necessarily free. A food can be labeled this
way even if it contains .5 g of fat per serving. So with some tempting
foods it is easy to have more than one serving and ingest too much
trans-fat. A perfect example is non-dairy whipped cream—the label

may say *trans-fat-free*, but that's only if you have a 2-tablespoon serving. It's often hard to stop at just 2 tablespoons of whipped cream. No amount of trans-fatty acid is a good amount, but ideally, sticking to 1 percent of your total fat per day should be your limit. Only 10 percent of your fat should come from saturated fat.

- Have one soy food per day. In October 1999, the Food and Drug Administration (FDA) authorized the health claim that soy is associated with a lower risk for coronary artery disease. A minimum of 6 g of soy and ideally 25 g of soy protein per day is recommended.

- Add garlic to your food daily. Garlic may help lower cholesterol levels. (See Roasted Garlic Bulb in Chapter 8 Recipes for a great way to add this food to your diet.)

- Keep to your low-sodium diet to help control your blood pressure. A diet of less than 2 grams of sodium per day continues to be best for helping with blood-pressure control.

- If you are overweight, work with a renal dietitian on a weight-loss program that is safe for you to follow.

- If you smoke or use tobacco products . . . *quit now.*

CANCER

Not only can certain kinds of kidney disease be caused by cancer, treatments for cancer, such as chemotherapy or radiation, may *cause* chronic kidney disease. Since the vegetarian diet is naturally higher in cancer-fighting nutrients, vegetarianism will help keep your immune function stronger for cancer prevention and treatment. To maximize your nutrition needs for both cancer and chronic kidney disease, try to use as many fresh, organic products as possible. Among other advantages, organic foods are naturally grown or raised and are certified free of additives, hormones, pesticides, and preservatives. Avoid the use of processed types of vegetarian foods, such as meat replacements or packaged vegetable dishes with added preservatives. If you are using dairy foods, choose organic products.

Fruits and vegetables should also be organic if possible. According to the Environmental Working Group, the ten most contaminated fruits and vegetables are apples, celery, cherries, imported grapes, lettuce, nectarines, peaches, pears, strawberries, and sweet bell peppers. These especially should be eaten in their natural, organic form.

If you are receiving cancer treatment, now is not a time to lose weight. If you are losing weight unintentionally, work with a renal dietitian to help you plan an adequate amount of nutrients to prevent further weight loss.

LUPUS NEPHRITIS AND KIDNEY DISEASE

Some of the first studies on vegetarianism and kidney disease were on people with lupus erythematosus. Research showed that lupus complications could be delayed or prevented with a vegetarian diet.

In addition to following a vegetarian diet, therapeutic supplementation with omega-3 fatty acids is also recommended. Table 4.3 shows a list of good food sources of omega-3. The recommended dosage for lupus varies, but it ranges from 1–3 grams. Omega-3 fatty acids have to be metabolized in order for their final end products, called docosahexaenoic acid (DHA) and eicosapentaenoic acid (EPA), to be most effective. The main source of EPA and DHA is fish oil (originating from certain types of sea algae). These end products are what help reduce inflammation in such diseases as lupus. You can obtain your alpha linoleic acid (ALA) omega-3 fatty acids from plants, but this requires conversion to EPA and DHA, which is estimated to be only 10–30 percent efficient. If you choose to obtain your omega-3 from plant ALA, you should triple your food source. To achieve 3 g of omega-3, you should consume 3–9 g of ALA per day. You might also want to add black currant oil as it contains gamma linolenic acids, which help with the conversion of ALA to EPA and DHA. (See Resources in back.)

POLYCYSTIC KIDNEY DISEASE

Polycystic kidney disease is a hereditary form of kidney disease. Fifty percent of the people who have this disease never develop kidney failure.

TABLE 4.3. FOOD SOURCES OF OMEGA-3 FATTY ACIDS		
FOOD SOURCE	PORTION	OMEGA-3 GRAMS
Flaxseed oil	1 Tablespoon	7.1
Canola oil	1 Tablespoon	1.6
Coconut oil	1 Tablespoon	.8
Sunflower or safflower oil	1 Tablespoon	.2
Wheat germ	1 Tablespoon	1.0
Walnuts, black	3 oz	3.3
Walnuts, English	3 oz	6.8
Egg enhanced with omega-3 fatty acids	50 g	.6
Soybeans	3 oz	1.5
Chinook or pink salmon	3 oz	1.48
Halibut	3 oz	.4–1.0

However, because this disease can potentially progress to kidney failure due to cyst formation on the kidneys, diet can be one way to slow the risk. Most important is to avoid foods that can promote cyst formation, and second is to avoid factors that can increase your blood pressure, which can affect the progression of kidney disease.

Caffeine and alcohol can promote cyst formation and should be limited as much as possible. Some obvious sources of caffeine are coffee, tea, and cola. Less obvious sources are chocolate, Anacin, and Excedrin. Carefully read labels on food and medications to avoid excess caffeine.

A vegetarian diet can help slow the progression of polycystic kidney failure. Studies have shown that soy products in general are beneficial in polycystic disease. In addition, increasing the use of omega-3 fatty acids and following a high-potassium diet may also be beneficial. A high-potassium diet, with routine potassium blood tests, can usually be eaten if your GFR is greater than 20 cc/min and you have not had high potassium blood levels in the past. Fruits and vegetables are your best sources of potassium.

IGA NEPHROPATHY

IgA nephropathy is the most common form of glomerulonephritis (GN) in the world. It often affects men more than women, and of those affected, approximately 20–40 percent will develop chronic kidney disease. A great deal of controversy surrounds the benefits of diet in IgA nephropathy, in particular the use of omega-3 fatty acids and a low-antigen-content (LAC) diet.

Supplementation with a good balance of DHA and EPA in omega-3 shows a favorable outcome. At least 3 g per day is recommended, though some studies have used as much as 12 g per day. DHA is difficult to obtain from plant oils and should be supplemented by either a fish oil or microalgae supplement in the amount of 1.8 grams per day. (See Resources in back for suggestions on brands.)

The food lists for an LAC diet will vary. Most current research shows there are benefits from limiting, if not totally omitting, foods containing dairy, eggs, and gluten. Table 4.4 will help you identify good substitutes. The biggest challenge will be getting used to eating a gluten-free diet. (See Chapter 8 for meal plans and recipes specific to an LAC diet.) (See also Appendix D in back for gluten-, egg-, and dairy-free eating.)

TABLE 4.4. GENERAL GUIDELINES FOR LOW-ANTIGEN-CONTENT DIET		
FOOD GROUP	FOODS TO AVOID	GOOD REPLACEMENTS
Dairy	All dairy products made with cow's milk	Soy, rice, or almond dairy substitutes
Protein	Eggs	Dried cooked beans, nuts, tofu
Grains	Barley, bran, bulgur, croutons, graham, kamut, rye, seitan, spelt, wheat, wheat germ	Rice, gluten-free grains, pastas, and cereals, such as amaranth, millet, potato flour, buckwheat, quinoa
Miscellaneous	Beer, soy sauce, thickeners	Sparkling water, brown rice syrup, Bragg Liquid Amino Acids, xanthum gum

5

The Kidney-Diet Link

WHAT DIET HAS TO DO WITH THE KIDNEYS

Twenty million Americans have chronic kidney disease—two out of every nine adults. There are many causes of this disease, but whether it was brought on by diabetes, genetics, high blood pressure, or other reasons, what you eat or do not eat impacts your disease process. Until recently, vegetarianism was thought to have a negative impact on your kidney disease, but it is now considered an eating lifestyle that can help preserve kidney function.

When you have kidney disease, your body develops uremia, or the buildup of waste products (also known as BUN) in the blood. One of these waste products is urea nitrogen, a by-product of protein metabolism. If you eat too much protein, or a *low-value protein,* the urea nitrogen level will build up sooner. In addition, several minerals, including calcium, phosphorus, potassium, and sodium, that you take for granted in your food are not efficiently filtered from the body and this can affect your disease.

Even though your kidneys are no bigger than the size of your fist, they have many functions, such as controlling anemia, bone formation, and high blood pressure, and they also affect your blood vessels and heart. A large part of the function of the kidney and how it interacts with these factors is affected by what you eat.

HOW THE DIET IS DIFFERENT
FOR EACH STAGE OF KIDNEY DISEASE

Because everyone is affected in different ways by their kidney disease, it is highly recommended that you check with your physician on which minerals are important or are a concern for your specific medical conditions. Table 5.1 reviews the typical diet guidelines required for different stages of kidney disease.

TABLE 5.1. DETERMINING YOUR DIET NEEDS		
YOUR STAGE	YOUR GFR	YOUR RECOMMENDED DIET NEEDS
1	90 cc/min	Low sodium
2	60–89 cc/min	Low sodium
3	30–59 cc/min	Low sodium, low phosphorus, low protein
4	15–29 cc/min	Low sodium, low phosphorus, low protein, and low potassium
5	< 15 cc/min	Low sodium, low phosphorus, low potassium, high protein (fluid restriction only if on dialysis)

PROTEIN

To build new tissues and replace old damaged tissues, the body uses protein as the building blocks. Sources of protein from vegetables include beans, grains, legumes, lentils, soy, and meat substitutes. If you are lacto-ovo vegetarian, cheese, eggs, milk, yogurt, and other dairy products also provide quality protein. Animal proteins include fish, meat, and poultry. By balancing the protein in your diet, you can minimize your blood level of urea nitrogen, feel better, and delay some of the complications of your disease, while still maintaining the growth of your tissues.

PHOSPHORUS

One important function of the kidney involves bone health. When the kidney filtering begins to decrease, your body retains phosphorus. As the level of this mineral rises in your blood, calcium begins to be pulled from your bones. This is the body's natural way of trying to balance these minerals in your blood, but the process can also make your bones weaker. Recent research indicates that high phosphorus can contribute to heart and vascular disease as well. So, in addition to watching protein, you may need to limit phosphorus-containing foods, as a low-phosphorus diet may help slow down kidney damage and avoid these complications.

Phosphorus is found in almost all foods, but it is especially high in animal proteins, cheese, milk, and yogurt. (See Table 5.2.) Some plant-based proteins, such as beans and nuts, are also high in phosphorus. In addition, since the 1990s, a surge of phosphate food additives has almost doubled the amount of this mineral in the typical American diet. Excessive phosphates can be found primarily in processed foods; biscuit, pancake, and waffle mixes; and cola drinks, and many other bottled beverages, even bottled iced teas.

In order to control the phosphorus in your diet, limit the foods listed in Table 5.2 to one serving per day. Also try to curtail the ingestion of any foods with phosphate additives, which go by many names, including disodium phosphate, monosodium phosphate, potassium tripolyphosphate, sodium hexametaphosphate, sodium tripolyphosphate, tetrasodium pyrophosphate, and trisodium triphosphate.

Plant-Based Diet Does the Trick

Steven, a sixty-year-old man with unexplained Stage 4 chronic kidney disease, came in to see me for nutritional counseling. His diet had been high in dairy and animal protein, but after I explained how this type of eating could have negative effects, he was quick to cut down on his high-phosphorus foods and switch to a plant-based diet. Only one month after doing this, Steven got himself down to a more manageable Stage 3 kidney disease.

If you are Stage 4 or 5, limiting foods high in phosphorus may not always be enough to keep your phosphorus level in a healthy range, and you may require phosphorus binders. This medication, taken with food, binds up the extra phosphorus in your digestive track before it can enter your bloodstream, allowing it to pass out of your body through your stool.

There are many types of binders. Some of the more common ones are Fosrenol (lanthanum carbonate), Phoslo (calcium acetate), Renagel (sevelamer hydrochloride), Renvela (sevelamer carbonate), or that good old standby, Tums (calcium carbonate). There is also a slow-release niacin treatment that has worked for people who do not want to take traditional binders. Most start out with 250 mg of timed-release niacin and progress to a higher dose of niacin (up to 1500 mg), as needed, to help control phosphorus.

In order to avoid having to take large doses of binders, it will help to keep your high-phosphorus foods in Table 5.2 to a minimum and avoid processed foods with phosphate additives.

TABLE 5.2. HIGH PHOSPHORUS-CONTAINING FOODS

Limit yourself to **one** of the following foods per day to help keep the amount of phosphorus in your blood at a normal level.

Milk (8 ounces or 1 cup)	Nuts (2 ounces or $1/2$ cup)
Cheese (2 ounces)	Waffles: frozen or mix (2 squares)
Soy milk (16 ounces or 2 cups)	Pancakes: frozen or mix (2 medium)
Cottage cheese ($3/4$ cup)	Macaroni and cheese (8 ounces or 1 cup)
Ice cream ($1 1/2$ cup)	Bran cereals:
Instant pudding ($1/2$ cup)	All Bran ($1/3$ cup)
Homemade pudding (1 cup)	100 percent Bran ($1/3$ cup)
Custard (1 cup)	Bran Buds ($1/3$ cup)
Yogurt (8 ounces or 1 cup)	Bottled iced teas (8 ounces or 1 cup)
Dark colas (8 ounces or 1 cup)	Hawaiian Punch (8 ounces or 1 cup)
Pizza ($1/4$ of 12-inch pizza)	

CALCIUM

When following a low-phosphorus diet, you may not get enough calcium, as many foods high in phosphorus also contain calcium. Therefore, many people on a low-phosphorus diet require a calcium supplement. Your blood can be tested to see what your calcium level is and to determine what you need. However, do not start taking a calcium supplement without first talking to your physician because if you supplement yourself without checking, your level could get dangerously high. Vitamin D can also affect the calcium level (*see* Chapter 7).

If your calcium becomes too high, you should review your diet for hidden sources. These include antacids, like Tums or calcium carbonate, or fortified foods, such as aspirin, cereals, crackers, or juices.

SODIUM

Most people with kidney disease require a low-sodium diet. Normally, when you ingest the mineral sodium, your kidneys get rid of what your body does not need. When your kidneys are not working well, however, sodium may build up in your body, and this can, in turn, cause elevated blood pressure and fluid retention (edema).

The sodium in your diet comes from both the food you eat and the salt you add. Salt (sodium chloride) is 40 percent sodium, and you should limit using it on your food. Since all salts are the same, this includes sea salt and rock salt. All stages of kidney disease can benefit from modestly restricting sodium to 2–3 grams per day. This can be achieved by limiting many of the processed foods, such as canned soup, fast foods, frozen meals, pickles, processed cheese, seasoning salt, snack foods, some of the meat substitutes, and soy sauce. The DASH diet recommends a 2,400 mg sodium diet, which can help control blood pressure, a big problem in the progression of kidney disease.

For many people, an occasional high-sodium food is desirable. Table 5.3 gives examples of these high-sodium foods and how you can safely work them into your diet in limited amounts.

Keep in mind that when you start limiting how much salt you eat, foods may taste different—and often *better*. On average it will take three weeks to lose the taste for excess sodium in the food you eat and start to appreciate foods as they really are.

	TABLE 5.3. SODIUM CONTENT OF FOODS		
FOODS	**HIGH SODIUM***	**MEDIUM SODIUM****	**LOW SODIUM**
	Limit to once per week	*Limit to once per day*	*Can be used freely*
Meat and Protein Substitutes	Frozen bean and cheese burrito; Frozen meatless entrée; Processed meat, such as bacon, sausage, lunch meats	Canned meat substitutes; Deli meats; Garden-burgers; Tofu hotdog	Fresh fish, meat, or poultry; Tempeh; Tofu; Seitan
Fruits and Vegetables	Dill Pickle,1 medium; Sauerkraut, 1 cup	Olives, 10 medium; Instant mashed potatoes, $1/2$ cup	Frozen vegetables; Fresh fruits and vegetables
Grains	Noodle or pasta entrée made from a package, 1 serving	Biscuit, 1; Chips, 2 oz; Packaged cookies, cake, or pie, 1 serving; Saltines, 10	Cookies, cake, or pie, homemade; Unsalted crackers; Unsalted popcorn; Wholegrain bread
Misc.	MSG; Soy sauce, 1 Tbsp	Buttermilk, 1 cup; Canned soups, 1 cup; Cheese spread, 1 oz; Commercial salad dressings, 3 Tbsp; Ketchup, 3 Tbsp; MSG, 1 tsp; Salt, $1/4$ tsp; Seasoning salts that contain the word salt—i.e. onion salt	Bragg Liquid Amino Acids; Herbs and spices (see Table 5.4)

*Contain approximately 1,000 mg sodium   **Contain approximately 500 mg sodium

Commercial Low-Sodium Products

There are several low-sodium spice mixtures on the market to choose from, but you need to be careful in your selection. Avoid mixtures that list salt or sodium as one of the first four ingredients on the label. If you are on a potassium-restricted diet, avoid spices mixtures that list potassium chloride as one of the first four ingredients. Table 5.4 provides several options for herbs and spices. You can also purchase a variety of low-sodium products. (See Resources in back.)

TABLE 5.4. BLENDS AND OTHER SEASONINGS TO TRY INSTEAD OF SALT

Apple pie spice	Wine	Wright's liquid smoke
Bragg Liquid Amino Acids	Bell pepper flakes	Bouillon (salt and potassium free)
Cinnamon sugar	Celery flakes/leaves	Chili powder
Garlic	Curry	Fine herbs
Hot sauce	Honey	Horseradish (fresh)
Lemon (juice, peel)	Italian seasoning	Leeks
Onions, onion flakes or powder	Molasses	Mrs. Dash
Poultry seasoning	Pickling spice	Pimento
Vegetable flakes	Pumpkin pie spice	Sugar
	Vinegar	Watercress

POTASSIUM

As kidney failure progresses, you may need to watch your intake of another mineral, potassium. Normally, when you eat potassium, your kidneys get rid of what your body does not need. When your kidneys are not working well, however, they may not get rid of this excess potassium, so it builds up in your blood. Potassium is involved in muscle contraction, and if your potassium level goes too high or too low, your muscles can become very weak. The most important muscle this can affect is your heart, which can be dangerous. If this happens, you will require a potassium-restricted diet. However, this often does not occur unless your kidney function is less than 20 percent or you are requiring dialysis treatments. You should also be aware that some medications can cause a potassium buildup or retention and you should ask your doctor about this.

Potassium is found in all foods, but is most concentrated in fruits, vegetables, and juices. For that reason, these are the foods that need to be limited on a potassium-restricted diet. Table 5.5 lists these foods in categories of high, medium, and low amounts of potassium. When requiring a potassium-restricted diet, most people can do quite well limiting themselves to *one* of the high-potassium foods per day, no more than *two* from the medium-potassium foods, and no more than *three* from the low-potassium foods per day.

TABLE 5.5. POTASSIUM FOOD LIST
HIGH POTASSIUM (250–500 MG)

FRUITS

Apricots (3)	Nectarines (1)
Avocados ($^1/_4$)	Oranges (1)
Bananas (1)	Papayas ($^1/_2$)
Cantaloupe ($^1/_4$ of 5" diameter)	Prunes (5)
Dates (5)	Raisins ($^1/_4$ cup)
Figs (3)	Tangelo (1)
Honeydew ($^1/_4$ of 5" diameter)	Watermelon (6" x 1" slice)
Kiwi (1)	

VEGETABLES*

Artichokes (1)	Pumpkin ($^1/_2$ cup)
Black-eyed peas ($^1/_2$ cup)	Spinach, cooked ($^1/_2$ cup)
Lentils ($^1/_2$ cup)	Split peas ($^1/_2$ cup)
Nuts: all kinds ($^1/_2$ cup)	Tomatoes (1)
Parsnips ($^1/_2$ cup)	Tomato sauce ($^1/_4$ cup)
Potatoes ($^1/_2$ cup or $^1/_2$ of medium, or 10 French fries)	Winter squash ($^1/_2$ cup)
	Yams, sweet potatoes ($^1/_2$ c)

JUICES

Orange juice ($^1/_2$ cup)	Tomato juice, ($^1/_2$ cup)
Prune juice ($^1/_2$ cup)	V-8 juice ($^1/_2$ cup)

OTHER

Milk

MEDIUM POTASSIUM (150–250 MG)

FRUITS

Apple (1 small or $^1/_2$ large)	Peaches, canned ($^1/_2$ cup)
Cherries ($^1/_2$ cup or 15)	Peaches, fresh (1)
Fruit cocktail ($^1/_2$ cup)	Pears, fresh (1 sm. or $^1/_2$ large)
Grapefruit ($^1/_2$)	Plums (2)

VEGETABLES

Broccoli ($^1/_2$ cup)	Mixed vegetables ($^1/_2$ cup)
Brussels sprouts ($^1/_2$ cup)	Mushrooms, raw ($^1/_2$ cup)
Beets ($^1/_2$ cup)	Okra ($^1/_2$ cup or 10 pods)
Carrots ($^1/_2$ cup)	Peanut butter (2 tbs.)
Celery ($^1/_2$ cup)	Peppers (1 or $^1/_2$ cups)
Eggplant ($^1/_2$ cup)	Potato chips (unsalted) (10)

Greens, cooked: beet, chard, collard, mustard,turnip ($^1/_2$ cup)

JUICES

Apple juice ($^1/_2$ cup)	Grapefruit juice ($^1/_2$ cup)
Apricot nectar ($^1/_2$ cup)	Pineapple juice ($^1/_2$ cup)
Grape juice, canned ($^1/_2$ cup)	

LOW POTASSIUM (100–150 MG)

FRUITS

Applesauce ($^1/_2$ cup)	Pineapple ($^1/_2$ cup)
Blackberries ($^1/_2$ cup)	Plums, canned ($^1/_2$ cup or 3)
Blueberries ($^1/_2$ cup)	Raspberries ($^1/_2$ cup)
Cranberries (1 cup)	Rhubarb, cooked ($^1/_2$ cup)
Grapes ($^1/_2$ cup or 15)	Strawberries ($^1/_2$ cup)
Pears, canned ($^1/_2$ cup)	Tangerines (1)

*See potassium content of beans in Appendix B.

VEGETABLES	
Asparagus (4 spears)	Onions ($1/2$ cup)
Beans: green / wax ($1/2$ cup)	Peas: green ($1/2$ cup)
Bean sprouts ($1/2$ cup)	Radishes (5)
Cabbage ($1/2$ cup)	Rutabagas, cooked ($1/2$ cup)
Cauliflower ($1/2$ cup)	Soaked potatoes ($1/2$ cup)
Corn ($1/2$ cup)	Summer squash ($1/2$ cup)
Cucumber ($1/2$ cup)	Turnips ($1/2$ cup)
Lettuce (1 cup)	Water chestnuts (4)

JUICES	
Cranapple juice (1 cup)	Kool-Aid (1 cup)
Cranberry juice (1 cup)	Lemonade / Limeade (1 cup)
Crangrape juice (1 cup)	Peach nectar ($1/2$ cup)
Grape juice, frozen (1 cup)	Pear nectar (1 cup)
Hi-C /Fruit drinks (1 cup)	Tang (1 cup)

FAT

Fat often gets a bad reputation. From unwanted calories to heart disease, it has often been identified as the food culprit. It is true that excess fat remains a health hazard, but amidst this obsession with using fat-free food, the less publicized benefits of fats should not be ignored. With kidney disease, you need 15–30 percent of your calories from fat, and even if you have heart disease, high blood pressure, or a high cholesterol level, you should still have at least 10–20 percent of your daily calories come from fat.

Saturated, Polyunsaturated, and Monosaturated Fats

The key to eating fat is to eat the right kind. There are saturated, polyunsaturated, and monosaturated fats. While saturated fats are very plentiful, giving people the pleasure of enjoying cream sauces, desserts, pastries, or flavorful snack foods, these fats can play havoc with your health. A high saturated-fat diet can contribute to heart disease and possibly certain kind of cancers.

Certain unsaturated fats have had hydrogen atoms added to give them a longer shelf life. These fats, often labeled as partially hydrogenated oils, are also known as trans-fatty acids and are found in many processed foods. They are *not* health-enhancing and may contribute to chronic illness.

Monosaturated fats, known as omega-9 fats, though not essential, can be important to your health. These fats help reduce your low-density lipoproteins (LDL), the bad cholesterol. Decreasing LDL is important in decreasing your risk for heart disease. By substituting monosaturated fats like olive or canola oil for more harmful fats, you can be assured of a good mix of the right fats.

Essential Fats

Some types of fat are essential for health and must be ingested. Linolenic acid (omega-3) and linoleic acid (omega-6) are called essential fats for this reason. Omega-6 fats are commonly found in many vegetables oils—corn, safflower, and sunflower—and some fish. Omega-3 fats are far less available, however, because they are so unsaturated they cannot be used in cooking, plus they have a very short shelf life.

Omega-3 fats are beneficial in all types of kidney disease. Most research has focused on this nutrient as especially beneficial for treatment of heart disease and high triglycerides; they may also delay the progression of kidney disease, particularly IgA nephropathy and lupus nephritis.

Coldwater fish, such as wild-caught salmon, flaxseed and flaxseed oil, nuts (notably walnuts), soy milk, and tofu are good sources of omega-3 fatty acids. In order to offset the excess of omega-6 fats, mainly due to its inclusion in a lot of processed foods, it is important to make sure you restore balance by adding omega-3 to your diet. Avoiding processed foods while eating at least one serving of omega-3 fats a day is a very important part of making this happen. The use of omega-3 fatty-acid supplements may also be of benefit above and beyond a healthy diet. (See Chapter 7 for additional information.)

The right balance of fats can reduce some of the complications of kidney disease, such as high-fat (lipid) levels in the blood, a poorly functioning immune system, or other chronic illnesses. Table 5.6 summarizes these fats to help you make wise selections in your daily food choices.

TABLE 5.6. TYPES OF FAT IN YOUR DIET AND THEIR SOURCES
SATURATED FATS
Found in: butter, dairy products, ice cream, meats, milk, and coconut, palm, and palm kernel oils.
Cholesterol is a fatlike substance produced by the livers of all animals, humans included. Found in: beef, eggs, fish, milk products, pork, and poultry. Found only in foods of animal origin.
Found in: fried foods; hydrogenated fats; packaged cakes, cookies, and pastries; processed foods; stick margarine; and trans-fatty acids.
POLYUNSATURATED FATS
Omega-6 fats. Found in: corn, cottonseed, safflower, soybean, and sunflower, oils, whole grains.
Omega-3 fats. Found in: canola, flaxseed, and soybean oils; flaxseeds; walnuts; and soy products.
MONOSATURATED FATS
Omega-9 fats. Found in: avocado, canola, flaxseed, olive, and peanut oils.

CALORIES

In the early stages of kidney disease, achieving and maintaining a healthy weight can help control blood pressure, which can, in turn, protect you from a progression of this disease. In any diet change, you usually need to reduce the portion size of certain foods and eliminate foods you have been used to eating, replacing these foods with others that will help you achieve the desired healthy weight. The suggested meal plans in Chapter 8 can help you with this.

When your kidney function is low, you may lose your appetite and not feel like eating. Taste changes and some nausea may make food less desirable, and for this reason you need to make sure you are not losing pounds. Weight loss in kidney disease can depress your immune system and cause you to be more susceptible to infections and other illnesses. Be sure to add appropriate fats and use the maximum number of servings you are allowed in each group. If you are still losing weight, you may benefit from a nutritional supplement that supplies extra calories. This needs to be selected with caution based on your level of kidney function, as many of these products are high in phosphorus, potassium, and protein, which can be dangerous to your health. Because of this, you should consult with a registered dietitian to determine the most appropriate nutritional supplement for you.

Eating too many calories, on the other hand, can contribute to weight gain, and this is also a health hazard in chronic disease. If you are overeating or gaining too much weight, stick to the lower end of the servings in the food lists, and be sure to keep your fat servings to a minimum.

6

Making Your Diet Plan

PUTTING IT ALL TOGETHER

Putting your diet together may seem like a challenge, given all the nutrients discussed. Table 6.1 has been designed to facilitate this. It can help you identify the amount of protein you need per day, along with balancing food choices to keep your phosphorus, potassium, and sodium in a healthy range.

Table 6.1 has been broken down into phosphorus, protein, fruits and vegetables, breads and grains, fat, and miscellaneous foods. It has been further broken down into *good choices* and *slow down*—the latter being foods identified as less desirable because they have more concentrated amounts of hydrogenated fats, phosphate additives, and sodium.

PHOSPHORUS GROUP

Certain animal proteins, colas, dairy products, and processed foods are high in the mineral phosphorus. You should begin limiting your phosphorus foods when your kidney function is at Stage 3, *even if your blood level for phosphorus is normal*. Early on in kidney disease, too much phosphorus can stimulate your body to produce an excess of the parathyroid hormone, which can cause too much calcium to be pulled from your bones and ultimately cause bone disease.

You cannot eliminate all phosphorus in your diet, but you can limit

TABLE 6.1. YOUR DAILY DIET PLAN

Food Group	Good Choices and Serving Size	Slow Down
High Phosphorus (1 serving daily)	2 oz cheddar, mozzarella, or other non-processed cheese; 1 cup milk; 1 cup plain yogurt; $3/4$ cup custard; $3/4$ cup pudding	Commercial iced tea; Dark carbonated beverages; Dark colas; Hawaiian Punch; Processed cheese
Quality Protein (for individual recommended servings, see Table 5.2)	1 egg (whites are best); 4 oz tofu, firm; 6 oz tofu, silken or soft; 2 oz seitan; $1/4$ cup meatless ground meat; $1/3$ cup dry cooked beans (limit to 2 servings per day); 2 Tbsp peanut butter (limit to once per day); $1/4$ cup nuts, preferably flaxseeds, walnuts, or pumpkin; 1 cup soy milk; $3/4$ cup cottage cheese (limit once per day); 1 heaping Tbsp whey protein powder	Canned meatless meats; Processed vegetarian entrees
Fruits and Vegetables (5–6 servings daily)	$1/4$ avocado; $1/2$ cup cooked or fresh vegetables; 1 small fresh or $1/2$ cup canned fruit, or $1/2$ cup juice; $1/2$ cup low-sodium tomato or V-8 juice	Pickled vegetables, such as dill pickles or sauerkraut
Breads and Grains§ (6–10 servings daily)	1 slice bread§ (1 oz); $1/2$ cup rice§, noodles, or pasta; 1 10-inch flour tortilla§; $1/3$ cup quinoa; 1 cup cold cereal; 6 unsalted crackers	Bread products with obvious salt crystals; Instant rice or noodles; Prepared grain mixes; Processed cakes, cookies, pies; Salted chips
Fats (as desired)	1 Tbsp butter or trans-fat-free margarine; 2 Tbsp cream cheese, regular; 1 Tbsp oil—canola or olive preferred for cooking	Fats in commercially prepared food; Stick margarine
Miscellaneous Foods	Coffee/tea; Lemon juice, lime juice; Vinegar; *Cream mints; *Hard candy; *Honey; *Jelly beans; *Kool-Aid; *Lollypops; *Sugar/syrup; **Jam/jelly; **Popsicles; **Soda pop, non-cola	Salt; Salt substitutes

* Avoid these foods if you have diabetes, and discuss how to include them in your meal with a registered dietitian or certified diabetes educator.
**Use sugar-substitute alternative if you have diabetes.
§ Gluten-free alternative can be used.

the foods that are most concentrated in this mineral. Colas can be re-placed with ginger ale, Sprite, or 7-Up; bottled iced tea can be replaced with homemade iced tea. In limiting dairy, there are many replacements for milk, including almond milk, rice milk, soy milk, and non-dairy creamers. Almond milk, rice milk, and soy milk are preferable to the non-dairy creamers because they are lower in concentrated sugars and devoid of saturated fats. Table 6.2 lists some of the more common milk substitutes.

TABLE 6.2. MILK AND MILK SUBSTITUTES (8 OZ SERVINGS)

Product	Calories	Protein (g)	Fat (g)	Sodium (mg)	Potassium (mg)	Phosphorus (mg)	Phosphorus Group Equivalent*
Almond milk	60–90	.5–1	2–2.5	75–150	160–180	45–100	.25
Milk, 2 percent	121	8.1	4.7	122	377	234	1
Mocha mix	305	< 1	25	158	320	130	.5
Mocha mix, light	160	< 1	12	68	290	120	.5
Rice Dream, original	134	< 1	3	70	15	15	0
Soy milk, creamy	160–210	7–9	7	130–180	210–450	160	.5
Soy milk, light	90–130	4	2	95–130	100–200	100–125	.5

*see Daily Food Guide for Phosphorus

ALMOND MILK

Almond milk is made from ground almonds and water, and occasionally with vanilla. As with rice and soy milk, almond milk does not contain lactose and can be used in many recipes calling for milk. Depending on the brand you select, its nutrient content is very similar to rice milk.

RICE MILK

Rice milk is made from brown rice and safflower oil. It comes in two types, original and enriched. The original is lower in phosphorus and potassium and can be used freely in your diet. Rice milk can be used as a direct replacement for milk in cooking or baking. This product is found mainly in health food stores, but more frequently now, Rice Dream is stocked by grocery stores.

SOY MILK

Soy milk is made from soybeans. It is higher in protein than either non-dairy creamer or rice milk. Compared to non-dairy creamers, the *light* brands of soy milk have a lower fat content. Soy milk comes in original, vanilla, and cocoa flavors.
Caution: The cocoa flavors are high in potassium.

Soy milk can be used as a direct replacement for milk in cooking or baking (custards, soups, and white sauces), but not in pudding mixes. This product is available in grocery stores and health food stores.

NON-DAIRY CREAMER

Non-dairy creamers are made from vegetable oil instead of milk fat. Most non-dairy creamers contain phosphate additives, which are not a recommended choice with kidney disease. Make sure any non-dairy creamer you use is free of phosphate additives. These can then be substituted for half and half in most recipes.

COOKING WITH MILK SUBSTITUTES

Non-dairy creamers should be diluted in cooking, 3 parts water to 1 part non-dairy creamer. Rice milk and soy milk can be used as is in recipes requiring milk.

Note: Milk substitutes cannot be used in place of milk in all situations. For example, these replacements will not make sour milk. And since instant pudding needs the acid in milk that is not present in these products, pudding needs to be made from scratch if using any of the milk-substitute products.

QUALITY PROTEIN GROUP

The amount of protein you need will depend upon your level of kidney function and your body weight. At least 50 percent of your protein should come from the quality protein group. Table 6.3 will help you determine how many servings of quality plant or vegetable protein you will need every day, based on your level of kidney function and your weight, to meet all your protein needs. To complete your protein needs, your diet plan will include 25 grams of protein from fruits, grains, and vegetables.

KG	STAGES 1 AND 2	STAGES 3 AND 4	STAGE 5**	RECEIVING HD	RECEIVING PD
		TABLE 6.3. KIDNEY FUNCTION IN CHRONIC KIDNEY DISEASE (Quality Protein* Servings Needed per Day)			
40	2	2	**	3	3.5
50	2.5	2.5	**	4	6
60	3	3	**	6	7
70	5	5	**	7.5	8
80	6	6	**	9	10
90	7	7	**	10	12
100	8	8	**	12	13

HD = hemodialysis

PD= peritoneal dialysis

*See list of quality proteins in Table 6.1

**At this level of kidney function you should be followed by a registered dietitian who specializes in kidney disease

Vegetarian protein foods are easily divided into three groups: beans and legumes, meat substitutes, and soy proteins. The exception to this is seitan, which is a very concentrated, grain-based protein from gluten.

Beans and Legumes

This group of vegetable proteins offers fiber, isoflavones, and trace minerals. Many experts in the field of kidney disease consider that all beans have the same protein, phosphorus, and potassium content, but the nutrient content of beans does, in fact, vary. This means that, although you can initially treat all beans the same, if you start to have specific problems with potassium or phosphorus levels, you may need to be more specific about the beans and legumes you select. For example, if your potassium is high, you may need to limit adzuki beans and eat lentils instead. If your phosphorus is high, you may need to switch to more lupin beans. (See Appendix B in back for the nutrient composition of some common beans and legumes.)

Soy Proteins

Soy has become very popular in recent years. Most of these products can fit well into your diet. Soybeans, soy milk, soy nuts, tempeh, and tofu are all soy foods.

Tofu is a very inexpensive, easy, and nutritious way to include quality protein in your diet. Unlike meats, it takes on the flavor of whatever you cook with it. It is very low in phosphorus, potassium, and sodium. Since there are different kinds, learning to cook tofu can be a new experience for many.

Types of Tofu

- Firm. This tofu is dense, solid, and holds well in stir-fry dishes, soups, or on the grill. It is highest in protein.

- Soft. This is a good choice for recipes that call for blended tofu. It works well in Asian soups or milkshakes.

- Silken. This is a creamier type of tofu that works well in blended dishes, such as cheesecake or lasagna. It mixes well with sour cream to make a higher protein topping.

Tips For Using Tofu

- Add chunks of firm tofu to your soups or stews in place of meat or with meat.

- Mix crumbled firm tofu into meatloaf.

- Mash tofu with cottage cheese or sour cream and season to make a high-protein spread for toast or crackers.

- Make a tofuburger. Mash soft tofu, breadcrumbs, chopped onion, and seasonings together and bake or grill.

- Replace all or part of the cream in soups with silken tofu.

- Make (missing) egg salad with tofu chunks, diced celery, mayonnaise, and a dab of mustard (*see* Recipes in Chapter 8).

- Replace powered milk with tofu milk powder in recipes.

- Stir-fry cubes of tofu with ginger, oil, and a dab of soy sauce, blend into rice or noodles, or put in pita bread.

- Egg replacement—2 oz of mashed tofu = 1 egg.

If you do not have an allergy, intolerance, or sensitivity to soy, this is where you should get the bulk of your vegetable protein. Research is very promising for soy proteins as a way to slow protein loss through your urine, preserve kidney function, lower high blood pressure, and reduce the risks of heart disease. If you are one who does not tolerate unfermented soy, such as soy milk or tofu, very well, you might try different types of fermented soy products, such as tempeh.

Certain soy-based products that would be healthy for others are detrimental in kidney disease. These include natto, which is high in potassium; miso, which is packed with sodium (sodium and kidney disease are a bad mix); and soybeans, which are high in potassium and phosphorus. Even though occasional use of these foods would be acceptable, they should be discouraged on a regular basis.

Changes in Diet Stabilize Chronic Kidney Disease

Margaret, a sixty-eight-year-old woman, was referred to me for diet counseling due to a slight rise in her creatinine levels consistent with Stage 2 kidney disease. She was used to eating in restaurants where the meals were high in meat and salt. Though Margaret did not want to become a total vegetarian, she did start using more soy and she cut down on animal proteins and sodium. Four years later, her kidney function has remained stable, not progressing beyond Stage 2.

MEAT REPLACEMENTS— PROCESSED SOY-VEGETARIAN FOODS

Meat replacements are generally considered vegetarian foods made from a variety of plant sources. For many, these products look and taste a lot like meat. They mainly contain soy or soy isolates (soy broken down into its various parts and presented separately, considered by some an inferior method of obtaining the nutrients and not as effective as the whole together). These foods can also contain beans, grains, legumes, nuts, or seeds, and most work well in a kidney-disease diet, except they tend to be much higher in sodium than unprocessed sources of grains, legumes, soy, and non-meat-substitute foods. For several of these products, the phosphorus content is not known or is not analyzed by the manufacturer. However, if the food is low in beans or dairy, it is probably fairly low in phosphorus. Refer to Appendix D in back for a list of the more common meat substitutes and nutrient compositions that are most appropriate for people with kidney disease.

Meatless meat products are a great substitute for meat in casseroles, spaghetti sauces, stews, and tacos. Vegetarian burgers are a delicious replacement for hamburgers in grilling and barbequing.

Seitan

Seitan is a vegetable protein made from wheat gluten. It is firm, has a meaty texture, and works well in casseroles and stews as a replacement for meat. However, a diet very high in this protein would lack some amino acids and would not provide the balance of amino acids you need. But filling no more than one-half of your protein requirement with this type of food is acceptable.

Seitan can be homemade or can be bought in a mix. Homemade seitan is much lower in sodium, but it can be quite time-consuming to make. When selecting processed brands, make sure to check the label for sodium. Those containing less than 700 mg per serving are recommended.

Seitan can be grilled, sliced for sandwiches, or used a a meat replacement in stews and other casseroles.

Quality Animal Proteins

If you continue to eat some animal-based proteins in your diet, it is best to select those that have the least effect on kidney filtration. In order of preferences, the best proteins are egg whites, eggs, fish, poultry, and red meat (including pork). It is unclear why some proteins affect kidney filtration more than others. The best theory, based on several studies, is that certain amino acids are metabolized differently and, as a result, some of these amino acids have a more beneficial effect on kidney function and filtration.

FRUITS AND VEGETABLES GROUP

Fruits and vegetables are often given a bad reputation with kidney disease, mainly because these foods are high in potassium. But in spite of this, these foods are very important for your long-term health because they are high in many antioxidants, phytochemicals, minerals, vitamins, and fiber.

The key is to select fruits and vegetables that are highest in beneficial nutrients, while minimizing nutrients that are of concern. Most people with kidney disease do not need to start limiting their dietary intake of potassium until Stage 4. Have your potassium level checked regularly to determine that it is in the normal range. Often with kidney disease, your body's system for maintaining a normal potassium level in the blood does not work well. As discussed in Chapter 5, if you eat too much potassium, your body may not get rid of it and you can become very ill. If you do not eat enough potassium, or become ill with diarrhea or vomiting, your potassium level may go too low. Diuretics and certain blood-pressure medications are used to treat kidney disease, and these medications can also affect potassium balance.

If potassium imbalances are not corrected, the weakness can spread to the upper body. Some people describe an *achy* feeling like the flu. Further, if not treated, a high potassium level can cause heart irregularities and actually stop the heart. This is why potassium regulation is so important in all stages of kidney disease. Refer to Table 5.5 in Chapter 5 if you require more restriction in your potassium-containing foods. Also, using Table 6.1, Your Daily Diet Plan, in this chapter, select a variety of colors in fruits and vegetables. This will ensure you are getting a range of nutrients.

BREAD AND GRAINS GROUP

Grains are often thought to be a complement to a meal but are not a source of protein. According to the old standards for evaluating protein quality, grains used to be thought of as *incomplete*. Newer standards of evaluation, however, reveal that these foods can be very complete and can add quality protein if included in a mixed diet of other foods, such as beans, dairy products, or tofu. The problem with grains eaten alone is that they lack certain amino acids, but when mixed with other foods, they can be part of a balanced protein source. Studies on Indian tribes who lived only off millet showed they had an unbalanced protein profile. But when millet was mixed with other foods, the amino-acid profile became complete.

Not only are many grains high in protein, they have other beneficial nutrients that are important in your diet. Table 6.4 lists some of the better grains and their nutrient content. You'll note that rice and barley are some of the lower potassium grains, whereas quinoa is higher in potassium and needs to be watched if you require potassium restriction.

Grains are high in trace minerals. Since extra supplementation of trace minerals is not recommended in kidney disease, getting these trace minerals only from your diet lessens the risk of toxicity while providing you with their beneficial nutrients.

TABLE 6.4. NUTRIENT CONTENT OF GRAINS ($^1/_2$ CUP COOKED, OR 4 OZ PORTIONS)

GRAINS	CALORIES	PROTEIN (g)	POTASSIUM (mg)	PHOSPHORUS (mg)
Barley	100	3	128	42
Bulgur	75	3	65	35
Couscous	100	3	50	20
Millett	120	4	75	120
Quinoa	120	5	209	141
Rice, brown	100	5	153	151
Rice, white	130	5	60	70
Seitan	70	15	46	275

FATS GROUP

You need fat. Fat provides concentrated calories and fundamental nutrients to your diet. As mentioned in Chapter 5, there are good fats and not-so-good fats. Your body requires two essential (good) fats to stay healthy—omega-6 and omega-3 fatty acids. Omega-6 fats are very plentiful in most diets, found in such foods as cooking oils and margarines. Omega-3 fatty acids are less plentiful, but are critical to your health, especially when you have kidney disease. You should have at least one serving of these foods every day in the form of firm tofu, flaxseed, flaxseed oil, soy milk (not fat-free), or walnuts. In certain types of kidney disease, such as polycystic kidney disease or lupus, it is best to consume omega-3 fatty acids every day. Research has shown polycystic cysts can decrease with the use of omega-3 fatty acids. Kidney damage has been delayed in lupus nephritis when omega-3 fatty acids are increased.

Please be aware that flaxseed oil *should not be used in cooking.* It is a very perishable fat and, if heated, it will oxidize and taste bitter, in addition to turning from an antioxidant to a pro-oxidant. This is harmful to your health, which is not what you want.

If you are hungry or need extra calories, it may be important to add servings to the fat group so you do not lose weight. However, if you are gaining too much weight, you may want to minimize your fat choices.

LABEL READING

When it comes to labels on food products, you can get a little overwhelmed. You may ask yourself why some products have potassium or phosphorus listed and others do not. This because the law only requires a listing of *calories, protein, sodium, fat, cholesterol,* and *fiber* on a product label. It does not require any listing for *potassium* or *phosphorus.* As of this writing, however, dietitians are trying to change this. If you are wondering whether a certain food can be worked into your diet, Table 6.5 can be a helpful guide. Most products do list the dietary value (DV) percentage of a food. You can use this number to determine how much phosphorus or potassium a food has and how it might work into your diet needs.

TABLE 6.5. HOW TO READ A LABEL		
	POTASSIUM	PHOSPHORUS
Low	< 100 mg, 3 percent DV	< 50 mg, < 5 percent DV
Medium	101–200 mg, 3–6 percent DV	51–150 mg, 5–15 percent DV
High	> 300 mg, > 9 percent DV	> 150 mg, > 15 percent DV

The calculations in Table 6.5 are based on a DV of 3,500 mg for potassium and 1,000 mg for phosphorus. For example, if you find a cereal you want to try that does not list the mg of phosphorus on the label, but has a DV of 15 percent for phosphorus, you can calculate that 15 percent of 1,000 mg equals 150 mg, and you will know this is a higher phosphorus cereal. If you are trying to cut down on phosphorus, you may want to try another cereal with a DV of 5–15 percent, or try not to use the cereal with a DV of 15 percent as often. If you find an entrée that has a potassium DV of 9 percent (9 percent of 3,500 mg equals 300 mg), you will also know this is a lot higher in potassium. If you require a potassium restriction, you can count this as your one high-potassium food for the day.

Sodium and protein will be listed on labels in mg and grams. To find out how to work these foods into your diet, count all side dishes with a sodium content less than 150 mg as low sodium, and count all entrées with less then 750 mg of sodium acceptable to eat once daily. With protein, if it is an entrée, count every 7 grams of protein as one protein serving. Breads, grains, fruits, and vegetables will vary a great deal and have been averaged into your diet guidelines to make your plan easier to follow.

Nutrition Facts

Serving size: 3.5 oz (86g)
Servings Per Recipe 3

Amount Per Serving

Calories 78	Cal. from Fat 10

	% Daily Value*
Total Fat 1g	**2%**
Saturated Fat 0g	**0%**
Trans Fats 0g	
Cholesterol 0mg	**0%**
Sodium 831 mg	**35%**
Total Carbohydrate 13g	**4%**
Dietary Fiber 6g	**25%**
Sugars 0g	
Protein 4g	

Vitamin A 8%	Vitamin C 0%
Calcium 4%	Iron 8%

* Percent Daily Values is based on a 2,000 calorie diet. Your daily values may be higher or lower depending on your calorie needs.

	Calories	2,000	2,500
Total Fat	Less than	65g	80g
Sat Fat	Less than	20g	25g
Cholesterol	Less than	300mg	300mg
Sodium	Less than	2400mg	2400mg
Total Carbohydrate		300g	375g
Dietary Fiber		25g	30g

Calories per gram:
Fat 9   Carbohydrate 4   Protein 4

Typical Food Nutrition Label

WHEN YOU DON'T KNOW WHAT'S IN A FOOD

You may find food you want to eat where the nutrient information is not available to you. Here are a few ways to handle this.

• If it is a commercial product, you can try to call, email, or write the company for nutrient information. Often the company may have the information, but for some reason does not list it on the package.

- Break down the nutrients the best you can. For example, if there are high potassium items in the food, count it as a high-potassium food. If it is more a protein-containing food, you will need to estimate protein servings—most average portions will be 2 or 3 protein servings. If there is milk or cheese in the food, count it as a high-phosphorus food.

- If this is a food you want to eat regularly, you can have your potassium and phosphorus checked the day after you have eaten the food to see what your levels are reading. This is a lot easier to do if you are regularly getting blood chemistries done, or if you are receiving dialysis treatments, where blood draws occur more frequently.

7

Vitamins, Minerals, Herbs, and Other Natural Supplements

VITAMIN AND MINERAL SUPPLEMENTS

Over the years, vitamin and mineral needs for kidney disease have changed a great deal. You should take a vitamin supplement, especially if you are not eating well. However, your selection of an appropriate vitamin supplement is crucial in order to balance out which nutrients are needed in kidney disease and which are not. For example, vitamin A is not tolerated well in the later stages (4 or 5) of kidney disease if your GFR is less than 50 ml/min.

If your GFR is greater than 50 ml/min, you can use an over-the-counter multivitamin. If your GFR is less than 50 ml/min, a renal vitamin is recommended. These include Nephrovite, Renex, Nephrocap, Dialyvite, or Vital–D RX.

The amount of vitamin C you take should not exceed 100 mg, due to oxalate end-products in kidney disease that can lead to artery hardening. And vitamin E needs to be supplemented in the right form.

In addition to a multivitamin, the following supplements may be beneficial. (See Resources in back for information on suppliers.)

Vitamin B$_{12}$

Vitamin B$_{12}$ is plentiful in dairy and animal proteins. If you do not eat any animal products at all, you can run the risk of low B$_{12}$ stores. Deficient B$_{12}$ is often treated with an injection of B$_{12}$ for better absorption.

It may be best to have your B_{12} level checked to make sure you do not need a therapeutic injection of B_{12} to replenish your stores. The best way to obtain B_{12} if you do not eat any animal products is with fortified food products or a B_{12} vitamin supplement.

You cannot count on plant sources of B_{12} to meet your B_{12} needs. These are found in some fermented plant foods and algae, but the B_{12} from these foods is not available in sufficient amounts to meet your needs.

Coenzyme Q_{10}

Coenzyme Q_{10} is a vitaminlike substance and is thought to be of benefit for a number of medical conditions and chronic illnesses. Low levels can contribute to muscle weakness, and poor heart and immune function.

Co-Q_{10} is also advised if you are taking any statin medications, such as Lipitor (atorvastatin) or Zocor (simvastatin). While these medications block cholesterol production in your body, they also block the production of coenzyme Q_{10}. Either situation warrants supplementation of coenzyme Q_{10}, usually 50–200 mg daily.

Vitamin D

There are two types of vitamin D that become important in kidney disease. One is called 25-hydroxy vitamin D, also known as an inactive vitamin D_3 or D_2. The second is called 1,25-hydroxy vitamin D, also known as active vitamin D. Vitamin D_2 needs to be metabolized by your kidney to turn it into the active 1,25-hydroxy form. Both serve very important functions in your health. Vitamin D_2 keeps your immune system strong and may help in managing blood pressure and preventing cancer. It also aids in your parathyroid hormone (PTH) function. Your PTH helps regulate calcium and phosphorus in your blood, and it is mainly regulated by vitamin D. If the hormone gets overactive, you may need more D_2 or 1,25-vitamin D.

Vitamin D metabolism can change very early on in kidney disease. It is difficult for food sources to meet your needs for vitamin D on a low-phosphorus diet. As a result, it is important that you have a blood test to determine your vitamin-D level. If you are low in vitamin D, you will need additional supplementation beyond what you can obtain in food or a multivitamin supplement.

In order to determine what kind of vitamin D you need, your doctor will need to test your blood for 25-hydroxy vitamin D and also check your PTH. This will help determine if you need vitamin D_2 or D_3, 1,25-hydroxy vitamin D, or both.

Your blood level of 25-hydroxy vitamin D will determine the amount of vitamin D you will need. Low 25-hydroxy vitamin-D levels are treated with vitamin D_2 or D_3, also known as ergocalciferol or cholecalciferol.

Vitamin E

Some studies of vitamin E say it prevents the progression of disease, while others say it does not. The reason for this confusion is that most studies do not differentiate the types of vitamin E used. Vitamin E is a fat-soluble vitamin that exists in eight different forms. Alpha tocopherol (a-tocopherol) is the most active form in humans. It is a powerful antioxidant. Many of the studies that were done on vitamin E were done with a synthetic vitamin E called *dl-alpha* tocopherol, while the natural form is labeled *d-alpha* tocopherol. For a more beneficial effect of vitamin E in chronic disease, it is best to eliminate *dl* tocopherol and stick to the natural tocopherols. These include alpha, beta, gamma, tocopherols—all forms of vitamin E that are found in such foods as nuts, oils, and seeds.

The RDA for vitamin E is 30 IU, but studies suggest therapeutic doses of 400 IU or more. This is often difficult to obtain from food sources, and supplementation is usually needed for these therapeutic doses.

When supplementing with vitamin E, limit it to less than 400 IU per day and select supplements that contain a mixture of naturally derived tocopherols (the label should read d-alpha tocopherols, delta tocopherols, gamma tocopherols, or mixed tocopherols and tocotrienols). Since some studies do note more benefit from food sources of vitamin E, try to add at least one food containing vitamin E per day. This can be a vegetable oil, a fortified cereal, nuts, or seeds.

Calcium Supplements

With a GFR less than 50 ml/min, you may not be able to meet your calcium needs with diet alone. At this point, supplementing with 500 mg of calcium per day is recommended. Do not add more than 500 mg without having your calcium level checked.

Carnitine

L-Carnitine is a nutrient made from amino acids that is used by your body to help with energy production. Since abnormalities in carnitine production have been noted in chronic kidney disease, and since the best source of carnitine is animal products, a supplemental dose of carnitine is warranted. Studies vary concerning dosage, but 600 mg a day for maintenance should be adequate. Testing carnitine levels in the blood is the best way for you and your healthcare provider to determine your needs.

Iron

Iron metabolism can change very early on in kidney disease. Your doctor should be checking your blood routinely to determine your iron needs. Often, supplementation is required, but this should not be initiated until your iron stores are measured. You should always try to add good foods rich in iron to help keep your iron level as high as possible. These include iron-fortified cereals, dried cooked beans, and blackstrap molasses. Working these into your diet will prevent your iron stores from decreasing too quickly.

If you do require an iron supplement, you will find several types to pick from. Most doctors prescribe ferrous gluconate or ferrous fumerate. If these cause problems with constipation or stomach upset, you may want to try iron supplements such as polysaccharide iron, known as NuIron or Niferex, or a polypeptide iron such as Proferrin. It is best to obtain a prescription for these products.

Probiotics

Probiotics and prebiotics share a unique role in health and disease. Regularly eating foods with probiotics or prebiotics can enhance your immune system, decrease allergic reactions, and improve your digestion. Probiotics are live microorganisms that you eat to promote healthy bacterial growth in your intestine. Prebiotics are foods that help stimulate the growth of healthy bacteria in your system.

There are many types of probiotics, and the type you need will vary depending on what your health problems are. For overall general health, *lactobacillus reuteri* or *lactobacillus casei* is good. For more immune support, you might need *bifidobacterium lactis*. These can be found in high-quality yogurts. Make sure you check the label to confirm that these are in the yogurt you select. Do not assume all yogurts have the same probiotics. Because of your phosphorus restriction, you may need to limit yourself to just one serving of yogurt per day. Supplements of probiotics can also be effective.

You should not treat yourself with probiotics if you are immune compromised. Examples of this might be if you are undergoing chemotherapy, recovering from a kidney transplant, or have any other active infection. If you are uncertain, check with your healthcare provider.

Prebiotics are another way to build healthy intestinal flora. Prebiotics can be added to your diet, but be sure to include plenty of whole grains, garlic, and onions. In addition, when choosing foods from your diet plan, make sure you add fresh fruits and vegetables. Fiber supplements can also be added. (See Resources in back.)

Trace Nutrients

Trace nutrients are supplements required by the body in small amounts. To date, they have not been recommended as supplements in kidney disease because research is still limited on their function and questionable excretion. Since many trace nutrients come naturally in a plant-based diet, it is probably best for now to obtain these nutrients from a variety of fruits, vegetables, oils, and plant-based proteins.

Zinc

Since a primary source of zinc is from animal protein, it is important to make sure you obtain enough zinc in your diet. Other good sources of zinc are fortified cereals, legumes, and nuts, but these may be difficult to obtain in the amount you need, so taking a vitamin with a minimum requirement of zinc is best. If you have healing wounds or sores, you may require higher doses. You should be evaluated by a healthcare professional before adding more zinc supplements.

PUTTING TOGETHER YOUR INDIVIDUAL SUPPLEMENT PACKAGE

To supplement your vegetarian diet, you can follow the guidelines in Table 7.1.

TABLE 7.1. YOUR SUPPLEMENT PACKAGE

You Need	How Much	Exceptions
Multivitamin or renal vitamin supplement with zinc and B_{12}	See Resources in back	You may need higher doses of zinc or B_{12} if you are deficient or your levels are in the low normal range
Coenzyme Q_{10}	50–200 mg	You may require 200 mg if you are taking statin medication
Vitamin D	1000–3000 IU D_2 or D_3	Have your vitamin-D level checked to see if you need higher doses
Vitamin E	400 IU natural form	
Calcium	500 mg	Have your blood tested to determine higher dose needs
L-carnitine	600 mg	If tested and found deficient in carnitine, you may require IV carnitine to establish normal levels
Omega-3 fatty acids	1 gm per day	See lupus and IgA section for higher dose recommendations

HERBAL SUPPLEMENTS

When faced with kidney disease, you may feel frustrated with your inability to cure your disease. You may feel further frustration by the numerous medications that your physicians prescribe for you. Feeling a lack of control and/or fear in your care may cause you to want to try alternative treatments, such as herbal remedies or vitamin supplements to treat your disease naturally. Some may be of great help, but with some, it is wise to err on the side of caution.

There are many reputable manufacturers of herbal supplements, but there are also some manufacturers of herbal supplements that do not follow strict controls, so you need to make sure any herbal supplements you take are not going to harm your kidney function. Some herbs are high in potassium, others can cause an increase in your blood pressure. Still others may interact with medications prescribed to prevent kidney rejection after receiving a transplant.

Some of the most helpful herbs and supplements include: ginger for digestion, ginkgo for circulation, glucosamine sulfate for joint pain, and Kibow Biotics, a probiotic-type supplement that can help rid your body of urea waste products. St John's wort may be helpful as well, but *not* in combination with other anti-depressants.

Herbs and supplements that require caution include many Chinese herbs, creatine, skullcap, and yohimbe.

Work with a healthcare professional who is familiar with herbs. Resources for information can be an herbalist, a renal dietitian, or a physician who is knowledgeable about herbal remedies. (See Resources in back for suppliers of herbal remedies.)

8

Meal Plans

There are two meal plans here. The first, Table 8.1, is for people with non-IgA nephropathy kidney disease, and the second, Table 8.2, is a low-antigen-content (LAC) diet, which limits or totally omits foods containing dairy, eggs, and gluten, for those with IgA nephropathy.

BOLD foods: You can add these freely to provide extra calories, especially if you are losing weight or have a poor appetite. Although butter is a better choice for a spread, as it contains *no* trans-fatty acids, you can substitute trans-fat-free margarine.

TABLE 8.1. NON-IGA NEPHROPATHY KIDNEY DISEASE		
DAY 1		
50 GRAMS	60 GRAMS	70 GRAMS
BREAKFAST		
1 slice toast; **Butter**; $1/_2$ cup regular oatmeal; $1/_2$ cup diced peaches; $1/_2$ cup soy milk	2 slices toast; **Butter**; 1 cup regular oatmeal; $1/_2$ cup diced peaches; 1 cup soy milk	2 slices toast; **Butter**; 1 cup regular oatmeal; $1/_2$ cup diced peaches; 1 cup soy milk
LUNCH		
$3/_4$ cup tofu eggless salad; 2 slices bread; Leaf of lettuce; **Mayonnaise**; Apple	$3/_4$ cup tofu eggless salad; 2 slices bread; Leaf of lettuce; **Mayonnaise**; Apple	$3/_4$ cup tofu eggless salad; 1 $1/_2$ oz soy cheese; Leaf of lettuce; 2 slices bread; **Mayonnaise**; Apple

50 Grams	60 Grams	70 Grams
Dinner		
1 serving Lentil Loaf*; 1 serving Almost Mashed Potatoes* **Butter**; $1/2$ cup green beans; 1 cup berries with **non-dairy whipped topping**	1 serving Lentil Loaf*; 1 serving Almost Mashed Potatoes*; 2 slices bread; **Butter**; $1/2$ cup green beans; 1 cup berries with **non-dairy whipped topping**	1 serving Lentil Loaf*; 1 serving Almost Mashed Potatoes*; 2 slices bread; **Butter**; $1/2$ cup green beans; 1 cup berries with **non-dairy whipped topping**
Snack		
5–6 gingersnaps; $1/2$ cup soy milk	5–6 gingersnaps; 1 cup soy pudding	5–6 gingersnaps; 1 cup soy pudding

DAY 2

50 Grams	60 Grams	70 Grams
Breakfast		
1 cup puffed rice cereal; $1/2$ cup soy milk; 1 banana	$1 1/2$ cups puffed rice cereal; 1 cup soy milk; 1 banana	2 cups puffed rice cereal; $1 1/4$ cups soy milk; 1 banana
Lunch		
1 Gardenburger; 1 oz soy cheese; Hamburger roll; Green salad with 1–2 Tbsp low-sodium salad dressing	1 Gardenburger; 1 oz soy cheese; Hamburger roll; Green salad with 1–2 Tbsp low-sodium salad dressing	1 Gardenburger; 1 oz soy cheese; Hamburger roll; Green salad with 2 hardboiled egg whites and 1–2 Tbsp low-sodium salad dressing
Dinner		
Indonesian Fried Rice* with 1 cup rice; 1 slice bread with butter; $1/2$ cup steamed broccoli	Indonesian Fried Rice* with 2 cups rice; 1 slice bread with butter; 1 cup steamed broccoli	Indonesian Fried Rice* with 2 cups rice; 1 slice bread with butter; 1 cup steamed broccoli
Snack		
1 serving Patti's Berry Fluff*	1 serving Patti's Berry Fluff*	1 serving Patti's Berry Fluff*

DAY 3		
50 GRAMS	**60 GRAMS**	**70 GRAMS**
BREAKFAST		
1 cup oatmeal; **Butter;** 1/2 cup soy milk; 1 cup blueberries	1 cup oatmeal; **Butter;** 1/2 cup soy milk; 1 cup blueberries	1 cup oatmeal; **Butter;** 1 cup soy milk; 1 cup blueberries
LUNCH		
1/2 cup Hummus*; 1 full piece of pita bread; Celery and carrot slices	1/2 cup Hummus*; 1 full piece of pita bread; Celery and carrot slices	1/2 cup Hummus*; 1 full piece of pita bread; Celery and carrot slices
DINNER		
1 serving Tofu Nougats*; 1/2 cup steamed beet slices; 1 cup rice; **Butter**	1 1/2 serving Tofu Nougats*; 1/2 cup steamed beet slices; 1 cup rice; **Butter**	1 1/2 serving Tofu Nougats*; 1/2 cup steamed beet slices; 1 cup rice; **Butter**
SNACK		
Tropical Smoothie*	Tropical Smoothie*	Tropical Smoothie* with one heaping Tbsp whey powder

DAY 4		
50 GRAMS	**60 GRAMS**	**70 GRAMS**
BREAKFAST		
1 Protein Pancake* with butter topped with 1 cup strawberries	1 Protein Pancake* with butter topped with 1 cup strawberries	2 Protein Pancakes* with butter topped with 1 cup strawberries
LUNCH		
Large green salad with 3 oz of seitan; 2–3 Tbsp low-sodium salad dressing; Hard roll with **butter**	Large green salad with 1 hard boiled egg or 3 oz tofu, or 3 oz seitan; 2–3 Tbsp low-sodium salad dressing; Hard roll with **butter**	Large green salad with 1 hard boiled egg or 3 oz tofu, or 4 oz seitan; 2–3 Tbsp low-sodium salad dressing; Hard roll with **butter**

DINNER

1 serving Pasta with Silken Tofu*; Dinner roll with **butter**; Peach slice	1 serving Pasta with Silken Tofu*; Dinner roll with **butter**; Peach slice	1 serving Pasta with Silken Tofu*; Dinner roll with **butter**; Peach slice

SNACK

Bagel; 2–3 Tbsp cream cheese	Bagel; 2–3 Tbsp cream cheese	Bagel; 1 oz soy cream cheese

DAY 5

50 GRAMS	60 GRAMS	70 GRAMS

BREAKFAST

2 Corn Cakes* with syrup; 1/2 cup applesauce; **Butter**	3 Corn Cakes* with syrup; 1 egg; 1/2 cup applesauce; **Butter**	3 Corn Cakes* with syrup; 2 eggs; 1/2 cup applesauce; **Butter**

LUNCH

Couscous Taco*; Apple; Tofu Brownie*	Couscous Taco*; Apple; Tofu Brownie*	Couscous Taco*; Apple; Tofu Brownie*

DINNER

Lentil Loaf*; **1 serving Almost Mashed Potatoes**; 1/2 cup mixed vegetables; 1 dinner roll; **Butter**; Peach slice	Lentil Loaf*; **1 serving Almost Mashed Potatoes**; 1/2 cup mixed vegetables; 1 dinner roll; **Butter**; Peach slice	Lentil Loaf*; **1 serving Almost Mashed Potatoes**; 1/2 cup mixed vegetables; 1 dinner roll; **Butter**; Peach slice

SNACK

1 cup cornflakes; 1/2 cup soy milk	1 1/2 cups cornflakes; 1/2 cup soy milk	1 1/2 cups cornflakes; 1 cup soy milk

DAY 6

50 GRAMS	60 GRAMS	70 GRAMS

BREAKFAST

3/4 cup cream of rice; 1/2 cup rice milk; 1/2 cup raspberries	1 cup cream of rice; 1/2 cup rice milk; 1/2 cup raspberries	1 1/2 cups cream of rice; 1 cup soy milk; 1/2 cup raspberries

LUNCH

Vegetarian Pastie*; Medium carrot slices; Medium apple	Vegetarian Pastie*; Medium carrot slices; Medium apple	Vegetarian Pastie*; Medium carrot slices; Medium apple

DINNER

1 serving Oven Roasted Tofu and Vegetables*; 1/2 cup pasta	1 serving Oven Roasted Tofu and Vegetables*; 1/2 cup pasta	1 serving Oven Roasted Tofu and Vegetables*; 1 cup pasta

SNACK

1 cup sherbet	Tofu Shake*	Tofu Shake*

DAY 7

50 GRAMS	**60 GRAMS**	**70 GRAMS**

BREAKFAST

2 Homemade Tortillas*; 2 Tbsp cream cheese; 1 cup blueberries	3 Homemade Tortillas*; 3 Tbsp cream cheese; 1 cup blueberries	4 Homemade Tortillas*; 4 Tbsp cream cheese; 1 cup blueberries

LUNCH

1 cup Tofu Chowder*; 6 low-sodium crackers; 1 cup grapes	1 1/2 cup Tofu Chowder*; 6 low-sodium crackers; 1 cup grapes	1 1/2 cup Tofu Chowder*; 12 low-sodium crackers; 1 cup grapes

DINNER

4 oz Seitan*; 1/2 cup pasta; 1 cup steamed zucchini; 1 serving Cranberry Salad*; 1 dinner roll and butter	4 oz Seitan*; 1 cup pasta; 1 cup steamed zucchini; 1 serving Cranberry Salad*; 1 dinner roll and butter	4 oz Seitan*; 1 cup pasta; 1 cup steamed zucchini; 1 serving Cranberry Salad*; 1 dinner roll and butter

SNACK

1 cup puffed rice cereal; 1/2 cup soy milk	1 cup puffed rice cereal; 3/4 cup soy milk	1 1/2 cup puffed rice cereal; 1 1/2 cup soy milk

*See Recipes.

§ In addition to the estimated grams of protein listed, all meal plans are based on averages and are estimated to provide less than 2,500 mg sodium, 2,500 mg potassium, and 1,200 mg phosphorus.

TABLE 8.2. MEAL PLANS ADAPTED FOR LAC-D §§

DAY 1

50 GRAMS	60 GRAMS	70 GRAMS
BREAKFAST		
1 slice gluten-free (GF) toast; **Trans-fat-free non-dairy margarine or spread**; 1 cup oatmeal; $1/2$ cup diced peaches; 1 cup soy milk	1 slice GF toast; 2 Tbsp peanut butter; 1 cup oatmeal; $1/2$ cup diced peaches; 1 cup soy milk	2 slices GF toast; 2 Tbsp peanut butter; 1 cup oatmeal; $1/2$ cup diced peaches; $11/4$ cup soy milk
LUNCH		
$3/4$ cup tofu eggless salad; 2 slices GF bread; Lettuce leaf; **Mayonnaise, soy-based**; Apple	$3/4$ cup tofu eggless salad; 2 slices GF bread; Lettuce leaf; **Mayonnaise, soy-based**; Apple	$11/2$ cup tofu eggless salad; 2 slices GF bread; Lettuce leaf; **Mayonnaise, soy-based**; Apple
DINNER		
$3/4$ cup Curried Rice with Cauliflower, Bell Pepper and Green Onion*; $1/2$ cup green beans; 1 cup berries	$3/4$ cup Curried Rice with Cauliflower, Bell Pepper and Green Onion*; $1/2$ cup green beans; 1 cup berries	$3/4$ cup Curried Rice with Cauliflower, Bell Pepper and Green Onion*; $1/2$ cup green beans; 1 cup berries
SNACK		
Tofu Shake*	Tofu Shake*	Tofu Shake*

DAY 2

50 GRAMS	60 GRAMS	70 GRAMS
BREAKFAST		
2 tortillas made with gluten-free flour; 2 Tbsp peanut butter and **jelly**; Peach slice	2 tortillas made with gluten-free flour; 2 Tbsp peanut butter and **jelly**; Peach slice	3 tortillas made with gluten-free flour; 3 Tbsp peanut butter and **jelly**; Peach slice

LUNCH

Grilled sandwich with 2 oz rice cheese and 2 slices GF bread; 1 cup green salad with oil and vinegar dressing	Grilled sandwich with 2 oz rice cheese and 2 slices GF bread; 1 cup green salad with oil and vinegar dressing	Grilled sandwich with 2 oz rice cheese and 2$^{1}/_{2}$ slices GF bread; 1 cup green salad with oil and vinegar dressing

DINNER

Stir fry with 4 oz tofu and 2 cups rice; 2 cups vegetables; **Trans-fat-free non-dairy margarine**	Stir fry with 4 oz tofu and 2 cups rice; 2 cups vegetables; **Trans-fat-free non-dairy margarine**	Stir fry with 6 oz tofu and 2 cups rice; 2 cups vegetables; **Trans-fat-free non-dairy margarine**

SNACK

1 cup berries	1 cup puffed rice cereal; 1 cup soy milk; $^{1}/_{2}$ cup berries	1$^{1}/_{2}$ cup puffed rice cereal; 1 cup soy milk; $^{1}/_{2}$ cup berries

DAY 3

50 GRAMS	60 GRAMS	70 GRAMS

BREAKFAST

1 cup puffed amaranth cold cereal; $^{1}/_{2}$ cup soy milk; 1 cup blueberries	1 cup puffed amaranth cold cereal; 1 cup soy milk; 1 cup blueberries	1 cup puffed amaranth cold cereal; 1 cup soy milk; 1 cup blueberries

LUNCH

$^{1}/_{2}$ cup Hummus*; 2 Homemade Tortilla Shells made with gluten-free flour*; Celery and carrot slices	$^{1}/_{2}$ cup Hummus*; 3 Homemade Tortilla Shells made with gluten-free flour*; Celery and carrot slices	1 cup Hummus*; 4 Homemade Tortilla Shells made with gluten-free flour*; Celery and carrot slices

DINNER

1 Serving Tofu Nougats*; $^{1}/_{2}$ cup rice; $^{1}/_{2}$ cup steamed broccoli; **Trans-fat-free non-dairy margarine**	1 Serving Tofu Nougats*; 1 cup rice; $^{1}/_{2}$ cup steamed broccoli; **Trans-fat-free non-dairy margarine**	1 Serving Tofu Nougats*; 1 cup rice; $^{1}/_{2}$ cup steamed broccoli; **Trans-fat-free non-dairy margarine**

SNACK

1–1$^{1}/_{2}$ cup sherbet	1–1$^{1}/_{2}$ cup sherbet	1 cup soy milk pudding

DAY 4

50 GRAMS	60 GRAMS	70 GRAMS
BREAKFAST		
2 pancakes with gluten-free flour made with soy milk; Fruit sauce	3 pancakes with gluten-free flour made with soy milk; Fruit sauce	4 pancakes with gluten-free flour made with soy milk; Fruit sauce
LUNCH		
3 cups green salad with 1 cup canned chickpeas; 2–3 Tbsp low-sodium or oil and vinegar salad dressing; Rice cake; 2 Tbsp peanut butter	3 cups green salad with 1$\frac{1}{4}$ cup canned chickpeas; 1 oz cheese substitute; 2–3 Tbsp low-sodium or oil and vinegar salad dressing; Rice cake; 2 Tbsp peanut butter	3 cups green salad with 1$\frac{1}{4}$ cup canned chickpeas; 1 oz cheese substitute; 2–3 Tbsp low-sodium or oil and vinegar salad dressing; Rice cake; 3 Tbsp peanut butter
DINNER		
4 oz tofu grilled with marinade; 1 serving Almost Mashed Potatoes*; **Trans-fat-free non-dairy margarine**; Red pepper stir fry	4 oz tofu grilled with marinade; 1 serving Almost Mashed Potatoes*; **Trans-fat-free non-dairy margarine**; Red pepper stir fry	8 oz tofu grilled with marinade; 1 serving Almost Mashed Potatoes*; **Trans-fat-free non-dairy margarine**; Red pepper stir fry
SNACK		
1 Tofu Brownie*	1 Tofu Brownie*	1 Tofu Brownie*

DAY 5

50 GRAMS	60 GRAMS	70 GRAMS
BREAKFAST		
2 Corn Cakes* with **trans-fat-free non-dairy margarine**; $\frac{1}{2}$ cup applesauce	2 Corn Cakes* with **trans-fat-free non-dairy margarine**; 1 egg; $\frac{1}{2}$ cup applesauce	4 Corn Cakes* with **trans-fat-free non-dairy margarine**; 2 eggs; $\frac{1}{2}$ cup applesauce

Lunch

1 Couscous Taco* (made with quick-cooking brown rice); Tofu Brownie*; Pear, fresh	2 Couscous Tacos* (made with quick-cooking brown rice); Tofu Brownie*; Pear, fresh	2 Couscous Tacos* (made with quick-cooking brown rice); Tofu Brownie*; Pear, fresh

Dinner

Lentil Loaf*; 1$\frac{1}{2}$ cup rice; $\frac{1}{2}$ cup peas and carrots; 1 dinner roll; Peach slice	Lentil Loaf*; 1$\frac{1}{2}$ cup rice; $\frac{1}{2}$ cup peas and carrots; 1 dinner roll; Peach slice	Lentil Loaf*; 1$\frac{1}{2}$ cup rice; $\frac{1}{2}$ cup peas and carrots; 1 dinner roll; Peach slice

Snack

1$\frac{1}{2}$ cups puffed amaranth cereal; $\frac{1}{2}$ cup soy milk	1$\frac{1}{2}$ cups puffed amaranth cereal; $\frac{1}{2}$ cup soy milk	1$\frac{1}{2}$ cups puffed amaranth cereal; $\frac{1}{2}$ cup soy milk

DAY 6

50 Grams	60 Grams	70 Grams

Breakfast

Tofu Milk Shake*	Tofu Milk Shake*	Tofu Milk Shake*

Lunch

$\frac{1}{2}$ serving leftover Lentil Loaf*; 3 cups lettuce salad with 2–3 Tbsp low-sodium or oil and vinegar salad dressing	1 serving leftover Lentil Loaf*; 3 cups lettuce salad with 2–3 Tbsp low-sodium or oil and vinegar salad dressing	1 serving leftover Lentil Loaf*; 3 cups lettuce salad with 2–3 Tbsp low-sodium or oil and vinegar salad dressing

Dinner

Pasta and Silken Tofu*; 1 cup cubed pineapple	Pasta and Silken Tofu*; 1 cup cubed pineapple	Pasta and Silken Tofu*; 1 cup cubed pineapple

Snack

1$\frac{1}{2}$ cups sherbet	2 Protein Pancakes*; Trans-fat-free non-dairy margarine	2 Protein Pancakes*; 2 Tbsp peanut butter

DAY 7

50 Grams	60 Grams	70 Grams
Breakfast		
1 cup puffed amaranth cereal; 1/2 cup soy milk; 1/2 banana	2 cups puffed amaranth cereal; 1 cup soy milk; 1/2 banana	2 cups puffed amaranth cereal; 1 cup soy milk; 1/2 banana
Lunch		
4 oz grilled tofu; 2 slices gluten-free bread with lettuce and tomato; Peach half	4 oz grilled tofu; 2 slices gluten-free bread with lettuce and tomato; Peach half	8 oz grilled tofu; 2 slices gluten-free bread with lettuce and tomato; Peach half
Dinner		
Rice and Black-eyed peas*; 1/2 cup canned beets; 2 homemade tortillas*; Trans-fat-free non-dairy margarine	Rice and Black-eyed Peas*; 1/2 cup canned beets; 3 homemade tortillas*; Trans-fat-free non-dairy margarine	Rice and Black-eyed Peas*; 1 cup canned beets; 4 homemade tortillas*; Trans-fat-free non-dairy margarine
Snack		
Tropical Smoothie*	Tropical Smoothie*	Tropical Smoothie*

§ In addition to the estimated grams of protein listed, all meal plans are estimated to provide less than 2,500 mg sodium, 2,500 mg potassium, and 1,200 mg phosphorus.

§§ LAC-d recipes are calculated using LAC-d grain, egg and dairy substitutes (see also Appendix D in back for gluten-, egg-, and dairy-free eating).

9

Recipes

HUMMUS

YIELD: 4 SERVINGS

2 cups cooked garbanzo beans
$1/_4$ cup bean stock
$1/_4$ cup lemon juice
2 cloves garlic
$1/_2$ Tbsp soy sauce
3 Tbsp tahini
2 Tbsp parsley, chopped

Purée all the ingredients together and let them sit at least 30 minutes to let the flavors develop.

Per Serving

Calories	106	Sodium	135 mg
Protein	4 g	Potassium	250 mg
Total fat	4 g	Phosphorus	200 mg
Total carbohydrates	14 g		

TOFU NOUGATS

YIELD: 3 SERVINGS (4 OZ EACH)

1 tsp Bragg Liquid Amino Acids*
(a tamari substitute), plus 2 Tbsp water
$^1/_2$ cup cornflake crumbs
1 tsp seasoning (garlic powder, curry, paprika, or other spice)
12 oz extra-firm tofu, cut into $^1/_4$ inch slices
Vegetable oil for coating the baking sheet

Preheat oven to 350°F.

Pour the Bragg into a small bowl. In another small bowl, mix together the cornflake crumbs and seasoning. Dip the tofu into the Bragg, then into the seasonings. Place the tofu slices on a baking sheet, lightly wiped or sprayed with oil. Bake for 20 minutes, flipping once to brown both sides, or fry the coated tofu in a little oil until both sides are browned.

*Bragg Liquid Amino Acids is an all-purpose seasoning made from soybeans.

Per Serving

Calories	180	Sodium	276 mg
Protein	22 g	Potassium	200 mg
Total fat	10 g	Phosphorus	130 mg
Total carbohydrates	7 g		

VEGETARIAN PASTIES

YIELD: 6 SERVINGS

If getting enough calories is a problem, this is a dish for you. They are easy to freeze and reheat too.

3 cups all-purpose flour
$^1/_4$ tsp salt
$^1/_2$ tsp baking powder

1 cup butter

4 egg whites

2 tsp distilled white vinegar

3$^1/_2$ cups water

1 cup dry lentils

1 potato, chopped

2 cups frozen mixed vegetables

1 onion, chopped

1 Tbsp olive oil

$^1/_2$ tsp Bragg Liquid Amino Acids

Preheat oven 350°F.

Dough: Mix flour, salt, and baking powder together in a medium-size mixing bowl. Cut in butter. Stir in egg whites, vinegar, and $^1/_2$ cup water. Continue stirring until dough is moist enough to be formed into a ball (add more water if necessary). Form the dough into a large ball.

Filling: Bring the remaining 3 cups of water to a boil, add lentils, and continue to boil for 30–45 minutes, until lentils are tender. Watch the lentils and add more water if necessary.

Wrap the potato pieces in aluminum foil and bake them for 30 minutes in the pre-heated oven. When they have cooled, cut into smaller pieces and mix with the lentils and mixed vegetables.

In frying pan, sauté onions with oil. Stir the onions into potato, vegetable, Bragg Liquid Amino Acids, and lentil mixture.

Divide the dough into 6-inch round circles. Lay the circles on a flat, floured surface. Place about one cup of filling into the center of each circle. Fold the dough around the filling, seal the edges, and arrange the pasties on an ungreased cookie sheet. Bake for one hour in the pre-heated oven.

Per Serving

Calories	700	Sodium	459 mg
Protein	20 g	Potassium	650 mg
Total fat	34 g	Phosphorus	295 mg
Total carbohydrates	83 g		

SOUP

TOFU CHOWDER

YIELD: 8 SERVINGS

2 Tbsp oil

1 medium onion, chopped

3 carrots, chopped

3 celery stalks, chopped

2 cups water

2 cups soy milk or other milk substitute

$1/_2$ pound tofu, crumbled

$1/_2$ tsp black pepper

$1/_2$ tsp celery seed

1 medium potato, peeled and chopped

Sauté together oil, onion, carrots, and celery in 4–6 quart pot for 15 minutes. Pour in the water and milk. Add tofu, pepper, and celery seed. Bring to a boil. Add potato pieces. Simmer until the potatoes are soft.

Per Serving

(analyzed with soy milk)

Calories	130	Sodium	74 mg
Protein	6 g	Potassium	384 mg
Total fat	7 g	Phosphorus	91 mg
Total carbohydrates	13g		

MAIN COURSES

CURRIED RICE WITH CAULIFLOWER, BELL PEPPER, AND GREEN ONION

YIELD: 4 SERVINGS

$1/4$ cup ($1/2$ stick) butter or substitute

1 Tbsp fresh ginger, peeled and finely chopped

$11/4$ tsp curry powder

$1/2$ tsp grated lemon peel

2 cups small cauliflower florets

$1/2$ cup red bell pepper, diced

$1/2$ cup green onions, chopped

$11/2$ cups long-grain white rice

2 cups water

$1/4$ tsp salt

1 cup frozen peas, thawed

Melt butter in heavy large saucepan over medium heat. Add ginger, curry powder, and lemon peel. Stir 30 seconds.

Mix in cauliflower, bell pepper, and onions, then rice. Add 2 cups water and $1/4$ tsp salt.

Bring to a boil, stirring occasionally. Reduce heat to medium-low, cover, and simmer until water is absorbed and rice is tender, about 18 minutes.

Remove from heat. Mix in peas and season with pepper. Cover and let stand 5 minutes.

Per Serving

Calories	425	Sodium	315 mg
Protein	9 g	Potassium	401 mg
Total fat	16 g	Phosphorus	174 mg
Total carbohydrates	63 g		

INDONESIAN FRIED RICE

YIELD: 8 SERVINGS

2 cups of brown rice in 4 cups water

1 cup meatless ground meat, such as Morningstar

1 Tbsp fresh ginger, peeled and minced

1 Tbsp catsup

1 Tbsp tamari

1 onion, sliced in half moons

1 red pepper, cut in 1-inch squares

1 carrot, cut in thin matchsticks

1 cup celery, diced

1 green pepper, cut in 1-inch squares

2 Tbsp dark sesame oil

2 cloves garlic, minced

Heat a 2-quart pan and add the rice. Cook and stir over medium heat for 6–8 minutes, or until rice begins to pop.

Remove from heat, add hot water, being careful of steam. Cover pan, return to heat, reduce heat to low and simmer 30–40 minutes until rice is tender and liquid is absorbed. Turn out on a large platter to cool.

Mix and set aside meatless ground meat, catsup, and tamari. Microwave for about 2 minutes to heat through, or cook until thoroughly heated.

Heat wok or large skillet and add oil, garlic, and ginger. Add the vegetables and stir-fry over medium high heat about 5–8 minutes.

Add the meatless ground meat crumble and vegetables to the cooled rice. Stir to mix and heat through. Serve hot, topped with sliced green onions.

Per Serving

Calories	200	Sodium	175 mg
Protein	10 g	Potassium	425 mg
Total fat	5 g	Phosphorus	190 mg
Total carbohydrates	33 g		

OVEN-ROASTED TOFU AND VEGETABLES

YIELD: 4 SERVINGS

16 oz extra firm tofu, drained
3 Tbsp balsamic vinegar
2 tsp olive oil
2 Tbsp sugar
1 clove garlic, minced
$1/_2$ tsp oregano leaves, dried and crushed
1 sweet red pepper, quartered
1 medium onion, quartered
4 medium mushrooms, quartered
Chopped parsley for garnish.

Cut tofu in half vertically then horizontally. Drain on several layers of paper towels to remove as much liquid as possible. If desired, score surfaces to allow more marinade to penetrate the tofu.

Combine vinegar, oil, sugar, garlic, and oregano. Mix well.

Place the tofu and vegetables in a shallow baking pan, leaving space between pieces for even roasting. Brush with the vinegar mixture and let stand for 30 minutes. After 30 minutes, brush again and let stand another 30 minutes or longer. During this time, preheat oven to 500°F.

Bake the tofu, pepper, and onion for 30–35 minutes. Turn once halfway through the baking time.

Add mushrooms during the last half of roasting time.

Transfer to a platter and sprinkle with parsley.

Per Serving

Calories	130	Sodium	50 mg
Protein	8 g	Potassium	275 mg
Total fat	5 g	Phosphorus	180 mg
Total carbohydrates	16 g		

PASTA WITH SILKEN TOFU
AND EDAMAME

YIELD: 6 SERVINGS

This dish is great hot or cold.

15 oz container of silken tofu

$^1/_3$ cup parmesan cheese

Pepper

1 pound fusilli or other short pasta.
Use gluten-free pasta if following the LAC-diet

1 cup frozen edamame

$^1/_3$ cup mint, finely chopped

Blend tofu and parmesan together.

Bring a large pot of water to boil and cook the pasta until al dente, as indicated on the package. Add the edamame to the pot for the final minute of pasta cooking time.

Drain pasta and edamame, reserving 1 cup of the cooking water. Add pasta to the bowl with the cheese mixture and $^1/_2$ of the reserved cooking water. Stir.

If the mixture is too dry, add more water 1 Tbsp at a time until creamy. Stir in the mint, season with pepper, and serve immediately.

Per Serving

Calories	415	Sodium	103 mg
Protein	22 g	Potassium	588 mg
Total fat	9 g	Phosphorus	340 mg
Total carbohydrates	61 g		

VEGETABLE DISHES

ALMOST MASHED POTATOES

YIELD: 6 SERVINGS

6 cups cauliflower (1 medium head)
4 oz cream cheese, or substitute
1 tsp garlic powder
$1/2$ tsp black pepper
1 tsp Worcestershire sauce

Cut cauliflower into pieces and rinse with water.

Place cauliflower pieces in a microwave-safe dish, cover, and cook on high for 8–10 minutes. Or place cauliflower in a steamer over 1 inch of water. Bring to a boil, cover, and steam for 8–10 minutes or until tender. Cool slightly.

Carefully place hot cauliflower into a food processor and blend until smooth.

Add cream cheese, garlic, and pepper. Blend to combine all of the ingredients.

Remove from the food processor and serve hot.

Per Serving

Calories	94	Sodium	76 mg
Protein	3 g	Potassium	198 mg
Total fat	7 g	Phosphorus	54 mg
Total carbohydrates	6 g		

CARROT CASSEROLE

YIELD: 6 SERVINGS

4 cups cooked, sliced carrots

$1^1/_2$ cups croutons

1 cup sharp cheddar cheese, shredded

2 eggs, beaten

$1/_4$ cup butter, melted

1 tsp Worcestershire sauce, or $1/_2$ tsp Bragg Liquid Amino Acids

Preheat oven to 400°F.

Place carrots in a buttered $1^1/_2$-quart casserole. Stir in croutons and cheese. Combine remaining ingredients and pour over carrot mixture.

Bake uncovered for 20 minutes or until brown.

Per Serving

Calories	330	Sodium	410 mg
Protein	17 g	Potassium	390 mg
Total fat	33 g	Phosphorus	295 mg
Total carbohydrates	15 g		

EGGPLANT CURRY

YIELD: 4 SERVINGS

This is great with rice or pasta.
You can add tofu for a little extra protein.
(Adapted from *The Candle Café Cookbook* by Joy Pierson and Bart Potenza.)

$1/4$ cup olive oil

2 medium onions, peeled and diced

4 garlic cloves, minced

1-inch piece of ginger, peeled and minced

1 jalapeño chili, diced

2 medium tomatoes, seeded and chopped

$1/2$ cup water

1 large eggplant, peeled and diced into 1-inch cubes

1 medium green or yellow bell pepper, seeded
and diced into $3/4$-inch pieces

1 medium red bell pepper, seeded and diced into $3/4$-inch pieces

1 tsp turmeric

1 tsp ground coriander

1 tsp ground fenugreek

1 tsp ground cumin

In a sauté pan, heat oil over medium heat. Add the onions, garlic, ginger, and jalapeño and cook for 5 minutes.

Add the tomatoes and cook for 3 minutes.

Add the water, eggplant, peppers, turmeric, coriander. Cook and stir occasionally for one hour.

Per Serving

Calories	165	Sodium	40 mg
Protein	2 g	Potassium	430 mg
Total fat	12 g	Phosphorus	63 mg
Total carbohydrates	15 g		

ROASTED GARLIC

3 garlic bulbs

Olive oil

Sea salt

Garlic roaster

Preheat the oven 400°F.

Cut the tops off of the garlic bulbs to expose the cloves. Peel off a few outer skins. Place the bulbs in the roaster. Drizzle olive oil over the top of the exposed cloves. Sprinkle with salt.

Cover and bake for 40 minutes.

Cool covered. You can store them in the refrigerator.

Per Serving—1 Clove

Calories	28	Sodium	117 mg
Protein	<1 g	Potassium	12 mg
Total fat	3 g	Phosphorus	5 mg
Total carbohydrates	<1 g		

BEANS AND LEGUMES

LENTIL LOAF

YIELD: 4 SERVINGS

1 small onion, chopped

1 tsp olive oil

2 cups cooked lentils, drained

$1/_2$ cup breadcrumbs or gluten-free alternative

1 cup rolled oats

$1/_2$ tsp thyme

$1/_2$ cup tomato puree

1 Tbsp vinegar

$1/_4$–1 tsp salt, or 1 tsp Bragg Liquid Amino Acids

Preheat the oven to 350°F.

Sauté the onion in the olive oil until soft. Add the sautéed onions to the remaining ingredients. Mix well.

Press the mixture into a loaf pan, cover with aluminum foil or a cookie sheet, and bake for 20 minutes. Uncover and bake for 10 minutes more.

Per Serving

Calories	280	Sodium	225 mg
Protein	14 g	Potassium	580 mg
Total fat	3 g	Phosphorus	300 mg
Total carbohydrates	50 g		

BLACK-EYED PEAS AND RICE

YIELD: 2 SERVINGS

1 cup uncooked rice
2 cups water
2/3 cup frozen black-eyed peas
1/4 cup onion, chopped
1 Tbsp oil
1 Tbsp low-sodium vegetable bouillon

Place rice and 2 cups of water in a saucepan. Add oil and bouillon. On high heat, bring to a rapid boil. When most of the water has boiled down (in about 5–7 minutes) put on lowest heat possible.

Meanwhile, stir-fry onion in oil until translucent. Rinse peas in fresh water, then add onion and peas to the pot of rice, stirring thoroughly.

Place a tight fitting cover on the pan and let simmer for 15–20 minutes.

Per Serving

Calories	300	Sodium	10 mg
Protein	10 g	Potassium	320 mg
Total fat	15 g	Phosphorus	480 mg
Total carbohydrates	95 g		

GRAINS AND FLOUR-BASED DISHES

COUSCOUS TACOS

YIELD: 8 SERVINGS (TACOS)

1 cup quick-cooking couscous
(for gluten-free use quick-cooking brown rice)
1¹/₂ cups boiling water
2 tsp extra virgin olive oil
¹/₂ ripe avocado, peeled and cut into chunks
¹/₂ medium tomato, seeded and diced small
¹/₂ cup red onion, chopped
8 corn tortillas
1 cup cheddar cheese, shredded, or soy cheese equivalent
2 cups iceberg lettuce, shredded

Place the tortillas in a 200°F oven to heat while you prepare the filling.

In medium bowl, combine couscous or rice, boiling water, and olive oil. Mix, cover, and let sit for 5 minutes. Remove cover and fluff with fork.

In another medium bowl, coarsely mash avocado. Stir in tomato and onions. (Any or all of the following can be added: a little lemon juice, hot sauce, chopped cilantro, salt, or pepper)

To assemble taco, spread warm tortillas with avocado mixture. Top with couscous or rice, cheese, and lettuce. Fold in half and enjoy.

Per Serving

Calories	250	Sodium	175 mg
Protein	9 g	Potassium	391 mg
Total fat	10 g	Phosphorus	190 mg
Total carbohydrates	31 g		

FRESH CORN CAKES

YIELD: 12 3-INCH CAKES

3 large ears fresh corn
1 large egg, or 2 oz mashed tofu
$1/_4$ cup unbleached white flour*
$1/_2$ tsp baking powder
Salt and pepper, to taste
Cooking spray or oil
*Gluten-free flour alternative can be used.

With a small, sharp knife, cut kernels from cobs (you should have about 2 cups).

In a food processor, pulse corn until chopped. Add remaining ingredients and process until smooth.

Let batter sit for 5–20 minutes. Stir batter before frying cakes.

Lightly spray or oil a large nonstick skillet or griddle. Cook heaping tablespoons of batter over medium-high heat until they begin to brown around the edges, about 2 minutes.

Flip and finish cooking, about 1 minute.

Per Serving

Calories	37	Sodium	27 mg
Protein	2 g	Potassium	83 mg
Total fat	1 g	Phosphorus	25 mg
Total carbohydrates	10 g		

FAJITAS

YIELD: 4 SERVINGS

4 whole-wheat fajita wrappers,
or four tortillas wrapped in foil
1 small red onion, chopped
2 medium garlic cloves, minced
2 bell peppers, seeded and sliced into strips
1 pound of seitan, cut into thin shreds
1 Tbsp chili powder
1 Tbsp soy-sauce substitute,
or $^1/_2$ tsp Bragg Liquid Amino Acids
2 plum tomatoes, peeled and finely diced
Low-fat sour cream

Place the fajita wrappers in a 200°F oven to heat while you prepare the filling.

Spray a medium skillet with olive oil cooking spray, add the onion and cook, stirring, over medium to low heat until softened slightly.

Add the minced garlic and bell peppers. Cook, stirring frequently, 5 minutes more.

Add the seitan, chili powder, and soy sauce or tamari. Lower the heat and simmer 5 minutes.

Place the fajita wrappers under a napkin to keep them warm and arrange the fajita filling on a small platter. Spoon a small amount of sour cream and tomato on top for garnish.

Per Serving (with Bragg)

Calories	325	Sodium	425 mg
Protein	30 g	Potassium	225 mg
Total fat	4 g	Phosphorus	80 mg
Total carbohydrates	35 g		

HOMEMADE FLOUR TORTILLA

Great for LAC Diet

YIELD: 1 SERVING

1 cup flour, can use any flour
1/8 tsp salt
1/2 cup water
2–3 tsp oil

In a bowl, mix the flour and salt. (For a puffier tortilla, add about 1/8 teaspoon baking power.)

Mix water and oil and add to dry ingredients. The dough should be soft, but not too sticky to handle. If needed, add a bit more water. Knead lightly. Pinch off pieces of dough to form balls (about 1 inch in diameter). Roll in a little flour to coat. Pat or roll into a flat circle about 1/8 inch thick. Repeat.

Heat a heavy skillet or griddle to medium, or 350°F. Do not oil. Place the tortilla on the hot pan and cook a few minutes, until it is lightly browned and starts to appear dry and develops a few air bubbles.

Flip and lightly brown on the other side. Cool, then place in a airtight container and store in the refrigerator, or freeze for later use.

Per Recipe

Calories	81	Sodium	38
Protein	3 g	Potassium	81 mg
Total fat	2 g	Phosphorus	69 mg
Total carbohydrates	15 g		

HOMEMADE SEITAN

YIELD: 8 SERVINGS

4 cups whole-wheat bread flour

4 cups unbleached white flour

6 cups water

Combine the 2 flours in a large mixing bowl. Mix the flour with enough broth to make a stiff dough. Gather into a ball and knead vigorously on a floured surface for at least 13 minutes.

Place in a bowl and cover the dough with cold water. Let it stand for $1/2$ hour or up to overnight in the refrigerator.

Pour off the broth and cover again with fresh cold water. Knead the dough under the water to wash out the starch and some of the bran. Pour off the milky white water and cover with fresh water. Keep washing and rinsing while kneading the dough until the water becomes almost clear.

Divide the dough in half, place the halves in a large stock pot and cover with 6 cups of broth. Bring to a boil and then turn down the heat and simmer for $1^{1}/_{2}$ to 2 hours.

Remove from the heat and set aside to cool. Slice the dough into steaks and place in large baking dish.

Cover with a marinade for at least 2 hours. (See recipe in Marinades, Sauces in this chapter.)

Seitan can be grilled over a charcoal barbeque, or even baked. If you are not using the seitan immediately, store it in the broth in the refrigerator, or drain and freeze.

Per Serving

Calories	430	Sodium	6 mg
Protein	14 g	Potassium	300 mg
Total fat	2 g	Phosphorus	275 mg
Total carbohydrates	91 g		

PROTEIN PANCAKE

YIELD: 1 SERVING

1 egg white

1/4 cup Quaker whole oats

1/4 cup low-fat cottage cheese or firm tofu

Mix vigorously and throw it on the skillet. Turn when needed. Cook both sides.

Per Recipe

Calories	100	Sodium	61 mg
Protein	7 g	Potassium	153 mg
Total fat	2 g	Phosphorus	109 mg
Total carbohydrates	14 g		

SCRAMBLED BREAD

YIELD: 1 SERVING

1 Tbsp butter or vegetable oil

1 slice of bread, broken into small pieces

2 egg whites

Melt butter or oil in a pan. Add bread and sauté until brown. Add remaining ingredients and cook until fluffy.

Per Recipe

Calories	220	Sodium	330 mg
Protein	10 g	Potassium	199 mg
Total fat	13 g		
Total carbohydrates	15 g		

SALADS

CHICKPEA SALAD

YIELD: 1 SERVING

$1/2$ cup cooked chickpeas

1 cup lettuce, shredded

$1/4$ cup carrots, shredded

3–4 slices of red/yellow bell peppers

$1/4$ cup canned mushrooms, no added salt

1 Tbsp onion, chopped

1 hardboiled egg, sliced

Place the shredded lettuce on a plate and layer with the sliced bell peppers, chickpeas, mushrooms, and onion. Top with the sliced boiled eggs.

Per Serving

Calories	275	Sodium	165 mg
Protein	14 g	Potassium	600 mg
Total fat	8 g	Phosphorus	270 mg
Total carbohydrates	39 g		

CRANBERRY CHERRY SALAD

YIELD: 8 SERVINGS

1 14.5 oz can pitted tart red cherries

1 3 oz package of cherry or raspberry gelatin

1 8 oz can jelled cranberries

1 3 oz package lemon gelatin

1 cup boiling water

1 3 oz package cream cheese, softened

$1/3$ cup mayonnaise

1 8 oz can crushed pineapple, undrained

$1/2$ cup non-dairy whipped cream

1 cup miniature marshmallows

Drain cherries, reserving juice. Set cherries aside. Add water to juice to measure 1 cup. Transfer to a saucepan. Bring to a boil.

Add cherry gelatin; stir until dissolved. Whisk in cranberry sauce until smooth. Add cherries and pour into an 1x7-inch dish. Refrigerate until firm.

In a bowl, dissolve lemon gelatin in boiling water.

In a small mixing bowl, beat the cream cheese and mayonnaise. Gradually beat in the lemon gelatin until smooth. Stir in pineapple.

Refrigerate until almost set.

Fold in whipped cream and marshmallows. Spoon this over cherry layer. Refrigerate until firm.

Per Serving

Calories	297	Sodium	156 mg
Protein	3 g	Potassium	114 mg
Total fat	11 g	Phosphorus	56 mg
Total carbohydrates	50 g		

EGGLESS EGG SALAD

YIELD: 3 SERVINGS

1 12.3 oz. package of firm tofu, drained

1 tsp each apple cider vinegar and honey

2 tsp mustard

$^1/_2$ tsp turmeric

2 Tbsp each celery and onion, diced

1 tsp parsley, chopped

Dash of paprika and pepper to taste

Crumble tofu into a small bowl. In a separate bowl, combine vinegar, mustard, honey, and tumeric. Mix thoroughly and pour over crumbled tofu.

Add celery, onion, parsley, paprika, and pepper. Mix thoroughly.

Refrigerate approximately 30 minutes to allow flavors to meld.

Per Serving

Calories	60	Sodium	100 mg
Protein	7 g	Potassium	350 mg
Total fat	30 g	Phosphorus	110 mg
Total carbohydrates	39 g		

MARINADES, SAUCES

BASIC SEITAN MARINADE 1

This recipes was adapted from The Candle Café Cookbook *by Joy Pierson and Bart Potenza. A wonderful cookbook and a MUST restaurant if you are ever in New York City.*

YIELD: 8 SERVINGS

2 tsp red wine vinegar

1 tsp molasses

Dash of garlic powder

$3/4$ cup water

1 cup virgin olive oil

$1/2$ cup Dijon mustard

8 cloves garlic powder

$1/2$ Tbsp of ground black pepper

1 tsp hot sauce

Put all marinade ingredients in a blender. Blend on high speed until well combined.

Per Serving

Calories	256	Sodium	376 mg
Protein	0 g	Potassium	12 mg
Total fat	27 g	Phosphorus	.5 mg
Total carbohydrates	.5 g		

BASIC MARINADE 2

This can be used on tofu or seitan.
(Adapted from the *Candle Café Cookbook.*)

YIELD: 8 SERVINGS

1 cup olive oil
1 cup lemon juice
2 garlic cloves, minced
$1/_4$ cup Agava Nectar
$1/_2$ cup parlsey
1 cup cilantro, finely chopped

Put all marinade ingredients in a blender. Blend on high speed until well combined.

Per Serving

Calories	282	Sodium	7 mg
Protein	<1 g	Potassium	31 mg
Total fat	4 g	Phosphorus	3 mg
Total carbohydrates	12 g		

TOFU ALFREDO SAUCE

1 pound silken tofu

1 clove of garlic, peeled

¹/₄ cup tahini

2 tsp Bragg Liquid Amino Acids, plus 2 Tbsp water (or ¹/₄ cup Soy Sauce Substitute [see below])

Blend all ingredients with 1 cup water in a blender or food processor until smooth. Transfer to a saucepan and cook for an hour over medium low heat, stirring occasionally.

Serve warm over pasta.

Per Serving (¹/₃ cup)

Calories	99	Sodium	118 mg
Protein	5 g	Potassium	178 mg
Total fat	7 g	Phosphorus	122 mg
Total carbohydrates	5 g		

SOY SAUCE SUBSTITUTE

Great substitute for LAC diet, or as
an alternative to high-sodium soy sauce.

4 tsp balsamic vinegar

2 tsp dark molasses

1 tsp ground ginger

1 pinch white pepper

1 pinch garlic powder

1³/₄ cups water

In a saucepan, over medium heat, stir together the balsamic vinegar, molasses, ginger, white pepper, garlic powder, and water.

Boil gently until the liquid is reduced to about 1 cup, approximately 15 minutes.

Per 2 Tablespoons

Calories	7	Sodium	1 mg
Protein	0 g	Potassium	40 mg
Total fat	0 g	Phosphorus	<5 mg
Total carbohydrates	2 g		

GLUTEN-FREE FLOUR MIXTURE

1 cup brown rice flour

2/3 cup tapioca flour

2/3 cup cornstarch

1 Tbsp xanthum gum

Blend these flours together and use as a replacement for wheat flour. This mixture can be used in making biscuits, pancakes, tortilla shells, or other recipes that call for flour. But be advised that it *cannot be* used to make seitan, which requires gluten-based flours.

Per Recipe

Calories	300	Sodium	96 mg
Protein	<1 g	Potassium	<10 mg
Total fat	4 g	Phosphorus	<1 mg
Total carbohydrates	67 g		

HERBED BAKED EGGS

YIELD: 3 SERVINGS

1 clove fresh garlic, minced

$1/_4$ tsp thyme leaves

$1/_4$ tsp fresh rosemary

1 Tbsp fresh parsley

1 Tbsp Parmesan cheese

6 eggs (before starting this recipe,
make sure your eggs are readily accessible)

3 Tbsp olive oil

$1^1/_2$ Tbsp butter

Ground pepper to taste

Toasted bread or English muffin

Preheat the broiler for 5 minutes and place the oven rack 6 inches below the heat.

Combine the garlic, thyme, rosemary, parsley, and Parmesan, and set aside.

Carefully crack 2 eggs into each of the 3 small bowls or tea cups (you will not be baking in these) without breaking the yolks.

Place 3 individual gratin dishes on a baking sheet. Place 1 tablespoon of oil and $1/_2$ tablespoon of butter in each dish and place under the broiler for 3 minutes until hot and bubbly.

Quickly, but carefully, pour 2 eggs into each gratin dish and sprinkle evenly with the herb mixture, then sprinkle liberally with pepper if desired.

Place back under the broiler for 5–6 minutes until the whites of the eggs are cooked (rotate the baking sheet once if they are not cooked evenly).

The eggs will continue to cook after you take them out of the oven. Allow the eggs to set for 60 seconds and serve hot on an English muffin.

Per Serving

Calories	340	Sodium	235 mg
Protein	14 g	Potassium	170 mg
Total fat	30 g	Phosphorus	230 mg
Total carbohydrates	5 g		

Egg Replacements

These are especially helpful for LAC diets where the flour can be replaced with a gluten-free flour. Each substitute below is equal to 1 egg. Use any one of these combinations in place of an egg in a recipe:

- 2 tablespoons liquid plus 2 tablespoons flour and $1/_2$ teaspoon oil
- 2 oz mashed tofu
- 1 Tbsp ground psyillium and 1 Tbsp water

DESSERTS

ANGELIC CAKE AND BERRIES

YIELD: 6 SERVINGS

1 cup lemon sorbet

1 tsp lemon zest

1 cup blackberries

1 cup strawberries

1 cup raspberries

1 store-bought angel food cake

Over low heat, melt sorbet with the zest of lemon in a small pan. Stir in the berries until they are coated with the sauce.

Cut the cake and pour the berries and sauce over the top.

Per Serving

Calories	216	Sodium	429 mg
Protein	4 g	Potassium	201 mg
Total fat	1 g	Phosphorus	165 mg
Total carbohydrates	50 g		

PATTI'S BERRY FLUFF

YIELD: 4 SERVINGS

This is a recipe created by one of my dialysis patients.
Everyone loved it, including the staff.

1 16 oz bag frozen unsweetened strawberries
(can substitute blackberries, raspberries,
or mixed berries)

1 Tbsp lemon juice

1 small (340 g) loaf of angel food cake

1 16 oz container Extra Creamy Cool Whip, thawed

4 Tbsp of Agava Nectar, amber or light
(can substitute 8 packets of Splenda)

Slice frozen strawberries in half. Place in a medium bowl. Sprinkle with lemon juice and toss. Drizzle with Agava or Splenda and lemon juice and toss.

Cover and place in the refrigerator until thawed (this can be done the night before).

Cut angel loaf into cubes. Place in a large mixing bowl with thawed berries. Fold mixture gently.

Add thawed Cool Whip and fold gently into cake.

Cover and refrigerate 2 hours.

Per Serving

Calories	425	Sodium	447 mg
Protein	5 g	Potassium	175 mg
Total fat	16 g	Phosphorus	28 mg
Total carbohydrates	69 g		

SECRET AUTUMN PIE

YIELD: 8 SERVINGS

Carrot pie might sound strange but it's delicious and is a great substitute for pumpkin pie, with the extra potassium. (Adapted from www.preparedpantry.com)

3 egg whites

$1/_2$ cup brown sugar

$1/_2$ cup granulated sugar

$1/_2$ tsp salt

2 cups cooked, pureed or mashed carrots

1 tsp vanilla extract

1 tsp ginger

$1/_4$ tsp cloves

$1/_4$ tsp mace

2 Tbsp flour

$1 1/_4$ cups Half and Half

Preheat oven to 400°F

In a large bowl, whisk egg whites until frothy. Add sugars and salt and stir until disolved. Add the rest of the ingredients and mix well.

Pour the filling into an unbaked pie shell (*see* recipe below). Bake for 45–50 minutes or until a knife inserted in the center comes out clean.

Per Serving

Calories	400	Sodium	209 mg
Protein	6 g	Potassium	119 mg
Total fat	20 g	Phosphorus	116 mg
Total carbohydrates	53 g		

HOMEMADE PIE CRUST

If you want to make your own pie crust, try this simple recipe. All you have to do is mix the ingredients together until a well-blended dough is formed and pat that into the pan.

1¹/₂ cups flour

¹/₂ cup vegetable oil

3 Tbsp sugar

3 Tbsp milk

SOY MILK PUDDING

YIELD: 2 SERVINGS

¹/₂ cup sugar

2 Tbsp cornstarch

¹/₈ tsp salt

1¹/₂ cups whole soy milk

1 tsp vanilla

In a saucepan, stir together the sugar, cornstarch, and salt. Slowly add the soy milk, stirring to prevent lumps from forming. Bring the mixture to a boil. Lower to simmer, stirring constantly for about 5 minutes, until mixture is creamy and thick.

Remove the pan from heat, stir in vanilla, and pour into dessert cups. Chill until mixtures sets.

Per Serving

Calories	300	Sodium	75 mg
Protein	5 g	Potassium	100 mg
Total fat	4 g	Phosphorus	60 mg
Total carbohydrates	75 g		

TOFU BROWNIES

YIELD: 12 SERVINGS

1 $^1/_3$ cups cake flour, or unbleached all-purpose flour
$^3/_4$ tsp baking soda
$^1/_2$ tsp cinnamon
1 12.3 oz package silken lite tofu
$^1/_4$ cup unsweetened applesauce
1 tsp canola oil
$^3/_4$ cup granulated sugar
1 tsp pure vanilla extract
$^1/_3$ cup cocoa powder
2 Tbsp walnuts, finely chopped, for garnish
(optional—increases the fat content per serving)

Preheat oven to 450°F.

Grease bottom and sides of 8 x 8-inch pan with vegetable shortening. Place waxed paper on greased pan bottom and grease top of paper.

In food processor, blend dry ingredients. Empty into small bowl; set aside.

Blend wet ingredients (except cocoa) in the food processor until smooth and sugar is dissolved. Add cocoa; process until smooth.

Add dry mixture all at once. Pulse to blend just until all dry ingredients are moistened.

Spread evenly into prepared pan. Sprinkle with chopped nuts.

Bake in oven for 20 minutes or until brownies spring back when touched lightly in center.

Let cool in pan for 15 minutes before turning out on cooling rack. Cool completely.

Per Serving

Without Nuts		With Nuts	
Calories	120	Calories	128
Protein	4 g	Protein	4 g
Total fat	1 g	Total fat	1 g
Total carbohydrates	25 g	Total carbohydrates	26 g
Sodium	25 mg	Sodium	25 mg
Potassium	79 mg	Potassium	72 mg
Phosphorus	50 mg	Phosphorus	44 mg

BEVERAGES

TOFU BREAKFAST SHAKE

YIELD: 1 SERVING

3 oz of firm or regular tofu

1/3 cup whole soy milk, rice milk, or almond milk

1 tsp vanilla

1/2 cup fruit (strawberries or other
low-potassium fruits are best)*

One or two ice cubes

Blend and enjoy

Per Serving (With Soy Milk and Strawberries)

Calories	144	Sodium	<50 mg
Protein	8 g	Potassium	200 mg
Total fat	8 g	Phosphorus	120 mg
Total carbohydrates	10 g		

*Banana is yummy in this, but counts as your one high-potassium food
for the day.

TROPICAL SMOOTHIE

YIELD: 1 SERVING

$1/2$ cup pineapple juice

$1/2$ cup milk substitute

1 scoop sherbet

$1/2$ tsp pineapple extract

$1/2$ tsp strawberry extract

1 Tbsp vegetable oil (optional, for extra calories)

Blend and enjoy

Per Recipe

Calories	430	Sodium	156 mg
Protein	8 g	Potassium	363 mg
Total fat	20 g	Phosphorus	135 mg
Total carbohydrates	85 g		

Metric Conversion Tables

98.6°Fahrenheit = 37°Centigrade

1 cc (cubic centimeter) = 1 ml (milliliter)

1 liter = 1,000 ml = 1 kg (kilogram)

1 liter = 2 pints = 1 quart

1 oz = 30 cc

8 oz = 240 cc = 1 cup

16 oz = 480 cc = 2 cups = 1 pint

1 lb. = 454 gm

1 kg = 1000 gm (grams) = 2.2 lb (pounds)

1 gm = 1000 mg (milligrams)

1 tablespoon (Tbsp) = $1/2$ oz = 30 cc

2 tablespoons = 1 oz = 60 cc

NUTRIENT ANALYSIS OF RECIPES (PER AVERAGE SERVING)

NAME OF RECIPE	CALCIUM (mg)	PROTEIN (g)	FAT (g)	CARBS (g)	SODIUM (mg)	POTASSIUM (mg)	PHOSPHORUS (mg)	VEGAN*	LAC DIET**
Hummus	106	4	4	14	135	250	200	Yes	Yes
Tofu Nougats	10	22	10	7	900	200	130	Yes	Yes
Vegetarian Pasties	700	20	34	83	459	600	270	No	No
Tofu Chowder	130	6	7	13	74	384	91	Yes	Yes
Curried Rice with Cauliflower	425	9	16	63	368	401	174	Yes	Yes
Indonesian Fried Rice	200	10	5	33	175	425	300	Yes	No
Oven-Roasted Tofu and Vegetables	130	8	5	16	50	275	180	Yes	Yes
Pasta with Silken Tofu	415	22	9	61	103	588	340	No	No
Almost Mashed Potatoes	94	3	7	6	76	198	54	No	Yes
Carrot Casserole	330	17	33	15	410	390	295	No	No
Eggplant Curry	165	2	12	15	40	430	63	Yes	Yes

*Recipes that say Yes in this column can be adapted to a vegan diet with milk, egg, or cheese substitutes.

** Recipes that say Yes in this column can be adapted to the LAC diet with flour, milk, egg, or cheese substitutes.

Name of Recipe	Calcium (mg)	Protein (g)	Fat (g)	Carbs (g)	Sodium (mg)	Potassium (mg)	Phosphorus (mg)	Vegan*	LAC diet**
Roasted Garlic	28	<1	3	<1	117	12	5	Yes	Yes
Lentil Loaf	280	14	3	50	300	580	300	Yes	Yes
Black-Eyed Peas and Rice	300	10	15	95	10	320	480	Yes	Yes
Couscous Tacos	250	9	10	31	175	391	190	Yes	Yes
Fresh Corn Cakes	37	2	1	10	27	83	25	Yes	Yes
Fajitas	325	30	4	35	675	250	80	Yes	No
Homemade Flour Tortilla	81	3	2	15	1	81	69	Yes	Yes
Homemade Seitan	430	14	2	91	5	300	275	Yes	No
Protein Pancake	25	2	1	3	16	40	32	No	No
Scrambled Bread	220	10	13	15	330	199	63	No	No
Chickpea Salad	300	21	12	40	165	900	395	Yes	No
Cranberry Cherry Salad	297	3	11	50	156	114	56	No	No
Eggless Egg Salad	60	7	30	39	100	350	110	Yes	Yes

*Recipes that say Yes in this column can be adapted to a vegan diet with milk, egg, or cheese substitutes.

** Recipes that say Yes in this column can be adapted to the LAC diet with flour, milk, egg, or cheese substitutes.

Name of Recipe	Calcium (mg)	Protein (g)	Fat (g)	Carbs (g)	Sodium (mg)	Potassium (mg)	Phosphorus (mg)	Vegan*	LAC Diet**
Basic Seitan Marinade 1	256	0	27	.5	376	12	.5	Yes	Yes
Basic Marinade 2	282	< 1	4	12	7	31	3	Yes	Yes
Tofu Alfredo Sauce	99	5	6	5	118	178	122	Yes	Yes
Soy Sauce Substitute	7	0	0	2	1	40	1	Yes	Yes
Gluten-Free Flour Mixtures	300	< 1	67	4	96	10	1	Yes	Yes
Herb Baked Eggs	340	14	30	5	235	170	230	No	No
Angelic Cake and Berries	216	4	1	50	429	201	165	No	No
Patti's Berry Fluff	425	5	16	69	447	175	28	No	No
Secret Autumn Pie	400	6	20	53	209	119	116	No	No
Soy Milk Pudding	300	5	4	7	75	100	60	Yes	Yes
Tofu Brownies	120	4	1	25	25	79	50	Yes	Yes
Tofu Breakfast Shake	144	8	8	10	< 50	200	120	Yes	Yes
Tropical Smoothie	430	8	20	85	156	363	135	Yes	Yes

*Recipes that say Yes in this column can be adapted to a vegan diet with milk, egg, or cheese substitutes.

** Recipes that say Yes in this column can be adapted to the LAC diet with flour, milk, egg, or cheese substitutes.

Glossary

Anemia. A condition where you have a low number of red blood cells in your body. It can make you tired and cold.

Artery. Blood vessel that carries blood from the heart to the tissues.

Artificial kidney (dialyzer). A mechanical device that removes waste from the blood and restores chemical balance in the body.

Blood access. The site that has been surgically established for use during dialysis.

Blood pressure. The pressure within the arteries. It reaches its peak when the heart beats and drops to its lowest level between beats.

Creatinine clearance. A test that measures the waste product creatinine in your blood and urine.

DASH Diet (Dietary Approaches to Stop Hypertension). This diet was developed specifically to help lower high blood pressure. The diet's key components are: 4 servings of fruit; 4 servings of vegetables; 7–11 servings of grains; 2–3 servings of low-fat dairy; nuts, fish, and poultry; very little red meat, sugar, or sugary drinks. Studies have shown that people with hypertension higher than 140/90 show reductions of 11 mg systolic and 5 mg diastolic on the DASH diet.

Deciliter. A measure of volume equal to one-tenth of a liter.

Dialysate (bath). The solution used in dialysis to remove metabolic waste products from the blood.

Dialysis. The process of maintaining the chemical balance of the blood by cleansing it when the kidneys have failed.

Dialysis access, hemodialysis access. Any device used to connect a person to dialysis. This includes fistulas, hemodialysis catheters, peritoneal catheters, and synthetic grafts.

Dry weight (tissue weight). A range of normal weight when no excess fluid is present. Your dry weight changes when your *tissue* body weight changes.

Edema. An abnormal accumulation of fluid in body tissues. You can check yourself for edema, or swelling, on your ankles, hands, face, or eyelids.

Erythopoietin (EPO). A hormone made primarily by the kidneys that tells your bone marrow to make red blood cells.

Fistula. A person's vein that is changed by joining it to an artery. The artery has a high blood flow and the vein has a lower blood flow, and this causes the vein to enlarge and the vein walls to become strengthened for hemodialysis access.

Glomerular filtration rate. A test to measure how well the kidneys are working. It measures how much blood filters through the glomeruli (the filters of the kidneys) per minute.

Graft. A tube or prosthetic vessel surgically implanted under the skin and joined to the patient's vascular system for access.

Hematocrit. The percentage of blood that is red blood cells.

Kilogram. A measure of weight. One kilogram equals 2.2 pounds.

Liter. A measure of volume. One liter equals 1.06 quarts.

Milli (m). A prefix used in the metric system meaning one-thousandth.

Milliliter (ml). A measure of volume. One milliliter equals one-thousandth of a liter.

Peritoneal catheter. A soft tube, about $1/4$ inch in diameter and 13–15 inches long, which is inserted into the peritoneal cavity through the skin of the abdomen, providing a small opening into the peritoneum through which dialysis can be placed.

Phosphorus binder. A medication taken with food that binds with phosphorus to block the phosphorus from getting into the blood. The bound phosphorus exits the body in the stool.

Protein. A nutrient used by the body to replace old or damaged tissues and to build new tissues, such as muscle and blood.

Uremia. The accumulation of waste products in the blood that the kidney normally filters into the urine.

Vascular. The blood vessels and the blood-transporting system in the body.

Vascular catheter. A synthetic tube or catheter inserted through the skin into a vessel to access the blood supply for hemodialysis.

Veins. The blood vessels that carry blood from the body tissues to the heart.

Waste products (metabolic end products). Chemicals produced by normal body functions that are not needed by the body.

Frequently Used Abbreviations and Chemical Symbols

BUN—Blood urea nitrogen	Kg—Kilogram
Ca—Calcium	Mg—Milligram
CC—Cubic centimeter	Na—Sodium
K—Potassium	PO4—Phosphorus

Blood Values Monitored
in Kidney Disease

Discussed below are the blood tests commonly monitored in kidney disease and the reasons you may have abnormal values. By understanding these blood tests, you are better able to manage your diet and, in turn, your health.

LAB TEST: POTASSIUM   NORMAL: 3.5–5.5 MMOL/L

If high:
- Too many fruits, vegetables, and juices in the diet
- If receiving dialysis, the dialysis solution may be too high in potassium
- Weight loss or internal bleeding
- Very high blood sugar

If low:
- Not eating well
- Vomiting or diarrhea
- Dialysis solution may be too low in potassium

LAB TEST: ALBUMIN   NORMAL: 3.5–5.5 G/DL

If low:
- Not eating enough protein
- Calorie intake too low
- Protein loss in urine
- Inflammation process, i.e., sickness, infection, etc.

LAB TEST: BUN (BLOOD UREA NITROGEN)
NORMAL: LESS THAN 100 MG/DL (IF ON DIALYSIS)

If high: (> 100 and on dialysis):
- Not dialyzing long enough
- Protein intake too high

NOTE: If you are not on dialysis, your BUN can also be high. But your physician will determine what that means to you.

LAB TEST: PHOSPHORUS   NORMAL: 2.5–5.5 MG/DL (IF ON DIALYSIS)
2.5–4.5 MG/DL (IF NOT ON DIALYSIS)

If high:
- Not taking enough phosphate binders
- Not taking binders at the right time
- Too many dairy products and other high-phosphate foods in the diet

If low:
- Taking too many phosphate binders
- Not eating well
- Vomiting or diarrhea

LAB TEST: VITAMIN D   NORMAL: 40–80 NG/ML

If high:
- Excess supplementation with D_2 or D_3

If low:
- Supplementation of vitamin D_2 or D_3 needed

LAB TEST: CALCIUM   NORMAL: 8.5–10.2 MG/DL

If high:
- Taking too much calcium or vitamin D

If low:
- Not taking enough calcium supplement or vitamin D
- Low magnesium levels

LAB TEST: PTH   **NORMAL: 35–70 PG/ML—STAGE 3**
                       70–110 PG/ML—STAGE 4
                       150–300 PG/ML—STAGE 4

If high:

- Not taking phosphate binders as prescribed
- Phosphorus is too high
- May need vitamin D supplementation

If low:

- Too much vitamin D
- May need a phosphate binder change
- May need other changes in medication

LAB TEST: CHOLESTEROL   **NORMAL: 150–200 MG/DL**

If high:

- Eating too many trans-fat foods
- Eating too many saturated-fat foods
- Not eating enough fiber food
- Above ideal body weight

If low:

- Not eating enough food in general

LAB TEST: HEMATOCRIT   **NORMAL: >36 PERCENT**

If high:

- Too many red blood cells
- Dehydration

If low:

- Blood loss
- Low iron stores
- Need erythropoietin or more erythropoietin
- Excess fluid

LAB TEST: CREATININE   NORMAL: .5–1.7 MG/DL

If high:

- Not enough dialysis
- Decreasing kidney function
- More muscle mass

If low:

- Low body mass

Composition of Nuts and Beans

	PROTEIN	CALORIES	POTASSIUM	PHOSPHORUS	POTASSIUM*
NUTS					
Almonds, raw 1/4 cup	6	167	156	148	Med
Black walnuts 1/4 cup	7	172	156	131	Med
White walnuts 1/4 cup	7	174	117	127	Low
Peanut butter, creamy 1 1/2 Tbsp	6	140	156	75	Med
DRIED BEANS					
Adzuki (b) 1/3 cup	5	70	370	115	High
Black beans (b) 1/3 cup	5	75	200	80	Med
Black-eyed peas (f) 1/3 cup	5	75	200	70	Med
Broadbeans (b) 1/2 cup	6	93	235	106	Med
Chickpeas (b) 1/3 cup	5	90	156	92	Med

	Protein	Calories	Potassium	Phosphorus	Potassium*
DRIED BEANS (cont.)					
Hummus 1/2 cup**	6	210	200	137	Med
Lentils (b) 1/3 cup	6	77	237	119	Med
Lupin (b) 1/2 cup	13	100	200	106	Med
Mung beans (b) 1/2 cup	7	95	200	140	Med
Navy beans 1/2 cup	7	130	330	140	High
Pinto beans 1/3 cup	3	45	180	75	Med
Red kidney beans (b) 1/3 cup	5	75	235	84	Med
Soybeans, green (b) 1/2cup	12	64	470	140	High
Soybeans, mature (b) 1/2 cup	14	75	470	200	High
White beans, small (b) 1/2 cup	8	130	414	150	High
Winged beans (b) 1/3 cup	6	84	156	88	Med
Yellow beans (b) 1/3 cup	5	85	200	108	Med

*See Table 5.5. Potassium Food List
**Foods with more than 200 milligrams of sodium; b=boiled, f=frozen

A one-ounce portion of meat has about 100 mg potassium and 65 mg phosphorus, while 1/3–1/2 cup of beans, or 1/4 cup of nuts ranges from 150–300 mg of potassium and 80–150 mg of phosphorus. This is a significant difference, yet careful adjustments in your fruit, vegetable, and starch servings will allow you to incorporate these foods into your daily diet plan.

Sheet for Tracking Your Progress

Date	
Labs	
BUN	
Creatinine	
Chloride	
Potassium	
Phosphorus	
Glucose	
A1C	
PTH	
Weight	
Blood Pressure	
Diet	
Phosphorus	
Vegetables	
Fruit	
Grains	
Protein	
Fat	

APPENDIX D

Product Information

	Size (g)	Protein (g)	Calories	Sodium (mg)	Protein Servings
PRODUCT INFORMATION FOR MEAT REPLACEMENTS					
Foods Per Serving*					
All American Classic Boca Burger	71	14	90	280	2
Big Franks, Kellogs	51	12	118	224	2
Blackbean Boca Burger	71	12	80	320	2
Chick 'n Grill Burger, Morningstar	71	13	100	360	2
Garden Vegan, Morningstar	71	10	100	230	1
Grilled Vegetable Burger, Morningstar	71	12	80	300	2
Tofu hotdog, Yves	38	8	35	300	1
Vegan Burger, Morningstar	71	13	70	280	2
Vegeburger, Kellog's Products	55	12	60	130	2
Vegetable Skallops, Kellog's Products	85	17	90	390	2

*Based on serving size on package

Note: Product information changes frequently. Always check labels.

See also Websites for Meat/Cheese-Replacement Recipes and Information in Resources.

PRODUCT INFORMATION FOR CHEESE REPLACEMENTS

Note: Product information changes frequently. Always check labels.

Foods Per serving*	Size	Protein (g)	Calories	Sodium (mg)	Protein Servings
Almond cheese, Galaxy cheese	28 g	7	50	190	1
Rice Vegan Cheese, Lisanatti	21 g	1	45	130	0
Tofutti cream cheese, Tofutti	2 Tbsp	1	85	160	0

*Based on serving size on package

See also Websites for Meat/Cheese-Replacement Recipes and Information in Resources.

Resources

Calorie and Protein Supplements

Ensure, Glucerna, Nepro, Promod, Suplena
Abbott Laboratories/Abbott Nutrition
625 Cleveland Avenue
Columbus, Ohio 43215-1724
Ph: 1-800-551-5838
Website: www.abbottnutrition.com

Arginine, Glutasolv, NV Renal, Resource
Nestlé Healthcare Nutrition
445 State Street
Fremont, MI 49413
Ph: 1-800-333-3785
email: cpsmail.nutrition@us.nestle.com
Website: www.nestle-nutrition.com

Fiber Resources

Benefiber
Novartis Consumer Health, Inc.
200 Kimball Drive
Parsippany, NJ, 07054
Attn: Consumer Affairs
Ph: 1-800-468-7746
Website: www.benefiber.com
Insoluble fiber supplement that can be added to beverages and other foods.

Clif Bar and Company
1610 5th Street
Berkeley, CA 94710-1715
Ph: 1-800-254-3227
Website: www.clifbar.com
Bars containing high-fiber ingredients.

Kashi Company
P.O. Box 8557
La Jolla, CA 92038
Ph: 1-877-747-2467
Website: www.kashi.com
A variety of cereal, meat replacements, and snacks high in fiber.

Unifiber
Alaven Pharmaceuticals
200 North Cobb Parkway, Ste 428
Marietta, GA 30062
Ph: 1-888-317-0001
Website: www.alavenpharm.com
Insoluble fiber supplement that can be added to beverages and other foods.

Herbal Remedies

American Botanical Council
6200 Manor Road
Austin, TX 78723
Ph: 1-800-373-7105 or
    1-512-926-4900
email: abc@herbalgram.org
Website: www.herbalgram.org
The council provides education using science-based and traditional information to promote responsible use of herbal medicine.

Consumerlab.com, LLC
333 Mamaroneck Avenue
White Plains, NY 10605
Ph: 1-888-502-5100 or
    1-914-722-9149
Website: www.consumerlab.com
This organization does laboratory evaluations on nutritional supplements.

Herb-Drug Interaction Handbook,
    3rd Edition
Church Street Books.
7 Church Street
Nassau NY 12123
Ph: 1- 518-766-4200 or 1-518-477-5771
email/website:
csbook@NYCAP.rr.com

Herb Research Foundation
4140 15th Street
Boulder, CO 80304
Ph: 1-303-4492-2265
email: info@herbs.org
Website: www.herbs.org
An in-depth resource for information about herbs.

Southcoast Health System
101 Page Street
New Bedford, MA 02740
Ph: 1-800-497-1727
Website: www.southcoast.org/library
Good information on drug interactions with herbal supplements.

United States Pharmacopeia
12601 Twinbrook Parkway
Rockville, MD 20852
Ph: 301-816-8223
email: uspverified@usp.org
Website: www.usp.org
For questions on USP dietary supplement verification program.

Vitamin and Mineral Supplements

Supplements for Stages 4 and 5 Kidney Disease

Dialyvite 3000,* Dialvite RX,*
    Dialyvite with Zinc
Hillestad Pharmaceuticals USA, Inc.
DialyviteDivision
P.O. Box 1010
Woodruff, WI 54568
Ph: 1-866-358-9773 or
    1-715-358-9773
email: info@dialyvite.net
Website: www.dialyvite.net
*Requires prescription from a doctor

RenaPlex, Vital–D RX
Nephro-Tech, Inc.
P.O. Box 16106
Shawnee, KS 66203
Ph: 1-800-879-4755
email: info@nephrotech.com
Website: www.nephrotech.com
Vitamin B-complex with zinc and folic acid.

Renax
Everett Laboratories, Inc.
29 Spring Street
West Orange, NJ 07052
Ph: 1-973-324-0200
email: info@everettlabs.com
Website: www.everettlabs.com
Renal-specific vitamin-mineral formula for elevated homocysteine levels, zinc levels, and oxidative stress in people with chronic kidney disease and undergoing dialysis.

Kebow Biotics
Kebow Biotechs, Inc
4629 West Chester Pike
Newtown Business Square
Newtown Square, PA 19073
Ph: 1-610-353-5130
Website: www.kibow.com
Probiotic supplement for nitrogen removal in kidney disease.

Supplements for Stages 1–3 Kidney Disease

CVS Daily Multiple 50 Plus
Rainbow Light
Eckerd Therapeutic M
Sundown Complete Multidaily
Eckerd Vita B
Theragam M Advanced

Nutrilite Daily
Available at most drugstores.

Omega-3 Fatty Acid Supplements

Advocare Omegaplex
Advocare International
Carrollton, TX
Ph: 1-972-478-4500
Website: www.advocare.com
Per soft gel: 300 EPA, 200 DHA

Carlson's Super Omega-3 Fish Oils
Carlson's Laboratory
Arlington Heights, IL
Ph: 1-847-255-1600
Website: www.carlsonlabs.com
Per soft gel: 300 mg EPA, 200 DHA

Coromega
Erbl, Inc
Vista, CA
Ph: 1-877-275-3725
Website: www.coromega.com
Per packet: 350 mg EPA, 230 mg DHA; Contains egg yolk

Kirkland Signature Natural Fish Oil
Costco Wholesale Corporation
Issaquah, WA
Ph: 1-425-313-8100
Website: www.costco.com
Per soft gel: 150 EPA, 100 DHA

Metagenics—EPA DHA Extra Strength
Metagenics
Ph: 1-800-692-9400
Website: www.metagenics.com
Per soft gel: 600 mg EPA, 400 mg DHA

Neuromins: Plant-Sourced DHA—
  Nature's Way Products;
  Non fish-based source
Martel Biosciences Corporation
Columbia, MD
Ph: 1-800-962-8873
Website: www.naturesway.com
Per soft gel: 100 mg DHA

Omega-3 700 Solgar—Vitamins
  and Herbs
Solgar Vitamins and Herbs
Leonia, NJ
Ph: 1-877-765-4274
Website: www.solgar.com
Per soft gel: 360 mg EPA, 240 DHA

Vitamin World—Naturally Inspired
  Super EPA Natural Fish Oil
Vitamin World
Bohemia, NY
Ph: 1-888-645-7135
Website: www.vitaminworld.com
Per soft gel: 300 EPA, 200 DHA; Contains gelatin

Websites for Gluten-, Dairy-, and Egg-Free Resources

Dietary Specialties. Website: www.dietspec.com (Ph: 1-888-640-2800)

Ener-G-Foods, Inc. Website: www.ener-g.com (Ph: 1-206-767-6660)

Gluten-Free Pantry. Website: www.glutenfree.com (Ph: 1-860-633-3826)

Gluten-free resources. Website: www.glutenfreeworks.com

Bob's Red Mill. Website: www.bobsredmill.com (Ph: 1-800-349-2173)

Information on gluten. Website: www.celiachealth.org

Websites for Low-Sodium Spices and Broths

Bakon Seasoning. Website: www.bakonyeast.samsbiz.com
  (Ph: 1-480-595-9370) • Bakon Hickory Smoke Style Seasoning.

Bragg. Website: www.bragg.com (Ph: 1-800-446-1990) • All-purpose
  seasoning made with soybeans and found in many health food stores.

Durkee. Website: www.spiceplace.com (Ph: 1-866-894-2865)

Lawry's Foods, Inc. Website: www.lawrys.com (Ph: 1-630-343-0240)

McCormicks. Website: www.mccormick.com • A selection of many spices.

Minors. Website: www.soupbase.com (Ph: 1-800-827-8328) • Flavoring
  ingredient for soups, sauces, gravy

Mrs. Dash. Website: www.mrsdash.com • Salt-free seasoning blends found
  in most grocery stores

Spice Hunter. Website: www.spicehunter.com (Ph: 1-800-444-3061)

Websites for Meat/Cheese-Replacement Recipes and Information

Boca Food. www.bocaburger.com (Ph: 1-877-966-8769)

Candle Café. www.candlecafe.com

Epicurious. www.epicurious.com

Galaxy Food. www.galaxyfood.com

International Vegetarian Union. www.ivu.org/recipes/

Kelloggs. www.kelloggs.com (Ph: 1-800-962-0120)

Lisanatti. www.lisanattichese.com (Ph: 1-866-864-3922)

Morningstar Farms. www.morningstarfarms.com (Ph: 1-800-962-0120)

Tavolo. www.tavolo.com

The Vegetarian Resource Group. www.vrg.org/recipes/

Tofutti. www.tofutti.com ((Ph: 1-902-272-2400)

Vegetarian Times. www.vegetariantimes.com/recipes/

Vegies Unite. vegweb.com/

Worthington Loma Linda. www.worthingtonfoods.com

Yves. www.yvesveggie.com (Ph: 1-800-434-4246)

References

A Clinical Guide to Nutritional Care in ESRD, 2nd Ed. Chicago, IL: American Dietetic Association. 1994.

American Dietetic Association, Vegetarian Practice Group. *Fact Sheet: Vegetarian Diet in Renal Disease.* Chicago, IL, 1998.

Anderson, J, Blake, J, Turner, J, et al. "Effects of soy protein on renal function and proteinuria in patients with Type 2 Diabetes." *American Journal of Clinical Nutrition.* 68(suppl):1347–1353S, 1998.

Anderson, J. "Soy Protein Decreases Risk for Heart Disease and Kidney Disease. Health Benefit of Soy Products through the Life Span." Lecture 10/6/2000.

Avery-Grant, A. *Eating Meatless on Dialysis: A Guide for Adult Hemodialysis Patients.* Cleveland, OH: The Centers for Dialysis Care, Inc. (Ph: 1-216-229-1100).

Bernstein, A, Treyzon, L. "Are High-Protein, Vegetable-Based Diets Safe for Kidney Function? A Review of the Literature." *Journal of the American Dietetic Association.* 107:644–650, 2007.

Bradley, Rebecca. "Advanced Glycosylated End-Products." *Renal Forum.* 5–6, Winter 1997.

Brookhyser, J. "Cooking with Tofu." *American Association of Kidney Patients: New Beginnings* (Formerly: *Renal Life*). 7, Winter 1999.

Brookhyser, J. "Omega-3 Fatty Acids." *Journal of Renal Nutrition.* 16:3.e7-e10. www.jrnjournal.org 2006.

Campion, E. "Why Unconventional Medicine?" *New England Journal of Medicine.* 328:282–283, 1993.

139

Coppa, R, Babola, B, Roleano, C, et al. "Dietary Gluten and Primary IgA Nephropathy." *New England Journal of Medicine.* 35 (18):1167–1168, 1986.

Cockcroft, DW, Gault, MH. "Predictor of creatinine clearance from serum creatinine." *Nephron.* 16(1):31–41, 1976.

Cupisti, A, Morelli, E, Meola, M, et al. "Vegetarian Diet Altered with Conventional Low-Protein Diet for Patients with Chronic Renal Failure." *Journal of Renal Nutrition.* 12(1):32–37, 2002.

D'Amico, G, Gentile, M, Manna, G, et al. "Effects of Vegetarian Soy Diet on Hyperlipidemia in Nephrotic Syndrome." *The Lancet.* 339:1131–1134, 1992.

D-Amico, G, Gentile, M. "Influence of Diet on Lipid Abnormalities in Human Renal Disease." *American Journal of Kidney Disease.* 22(1):151–157, 1993.

Dietitians' Association of Australia. "Evidence-Based Practice Guidelines for the Nutritional Management of Chronic Kidney Disease." *Nutrition and Dietetics.* 63(Supp 2):S35–S45, 2006.

Donadio, J. "The Role of Omega-3 Fatty Acids in the Practice of Nephrology." Presented at National Kidney Foundation Clinical Nephrology Meeting, 2002.

Douglas, L, Sanders, M. "Probiotics and Prebiotics in Dietetics Practice." *Journal of the American Dietetic Association.* 108(3):510–521, 2008.

Eisenberg, D, Davis, R, Ettner, S, et al. "Trend in Alternative Medicine Use in the US. (1990–1997)" *Journal of the American Medical Association.* 280: 1569–1575, November 11, 1998.

Ernst, E. "Harmless Herbs? A review of recent literature." *The American Journal of Medicine.* 104:170–178, 1998.

Fair, D, Ogborn, M, Weller, H, et al. "Dietary Soy Protein Attentuates Renal Disease Progression After 1 and 3 Weeks in Han:SPRD-*cy* Weaning Rats." *Journal of Renal Nutrition.* 134(6):1505–1507, June 2004.

Fanti, P. "Soyfoods in Chronic Renal Disease." Third Annual Soyfoods Symposium Proceedings:1–5, 1999.

Fanti, P. "Soyfoods in Chronic Renal Disease." Third Annual Soyfoods Symposium Proceedings, June 1999. Gallup, G, Gallup GH. The Gallup Poll. Public Opinion 1996. *Scholarly Resources.* Wilmington, DE, 1997.

Ferri, C, Puccini, R, Longombardo, G. "Low-antigen content diet in the treatment of patients with IgA Nephropathy." *Nephrology Dialysis Transplantation.* 8:1193–1198, 1993.

Ferri, C, Puccini, R. "Low Antigen Content Diet."

http://www.do.med.unipi.it/apher/write/diet.htm 2007.

Gianni, L, Dreitlein, W. "Some Popular OTC Herbals Can Interact with Anti-coagulant Therapy." *US Pharmacist.* 80–84, 1998.

Golper, T, Ahmad, S. "L Carnitine Administration to Hemodialysis Patients. Has Its Time Come?" *Seminars in Dialysis.* 5(2):94–98, Apr–Jun 1992.

Jones, G. "Expanding Role for vitamin D in Chronic Kidney Disease: Importance of Blood 25-OH Levels and Extra-Renal 1,Hydroxlase In the Classical and Nonclassical Actions of 1,25-Dihydroxyvitamin D3." *Seminars in Dialysis.* 20 (4):316–324, 2007.

Kopple, J. *Nutritional Management in Kidney Disease.* Baltimore, MD: Williams and Wilkens, 1997.

Kuhn, M. *Herbs, Drugs and the Body. Oldest and Newest Forms of Therapy.* Hamburg, NY: Medical Educational Services, 1999.

Messina, M, Messina, V. *The Simple Soybean and Your Health.* Garden City Park, NY: Avery Publishing Group, 1994.

Miller, L. "Herbal Medicinals and Selected Clinical Considerations: Focusing on Known or Potential Drug-Herb Interactions." *Archives of Internal Medicine.* 158, 1998.

Neustadt, J, Pizzorno, J. "Vitamin E and All Cause Mortality." *Integrative Medicine.* 4(1):1–16, Feb-Mar 2005.

NKF-DOQI, Nutritional Guidelines. New York: National Kidney Foundation, 2000.

Pagenkemper, J. "Planning a Vegetarian Renal Diet." *Journal of Renal Nutrition.* 5(4): 234–238, 1995.

Patel, C. "Vegetarian Renal Diet and Practical Applications." Renal Nutrition Forum. *Journal of the American Dietetic Association.* 219:(3), 2000.

Pellett, P. Protein Requirements in Humans. *American Journal of Clinical Nutrition.* 51(92):723–737,1990.

Practice Guidelines for Nutritional Care of Renal Patients, 3rd Ed. American Dietetic Associaton, 2000.

Richman, A, Witkosdi, J. "Herbs by the Numbers." *Whole Foods Magazine.* 20–28, 1997.

Rostoker, G. "Therapy of IgA Nephropathy." *Biodrugs.* 4:279–301, Apr 9, 1998.

Rundek, T, Naini, A, Sacco, R. "Atrovastatin decreases the coenzyme Q_{10} level in the blood of patients at risk for cardiovascular disease and stroke." *Archives of Neurology.* 61(6):889–892, 2004.

Soroka, N, Silverberg, D, Greemland, M, et al. "Comparison of a Vegetable Based (Soya) and an Animal-Based Low Protein Diet in Pre-dialysis Chronic Renal Failure Patients." *Nephron.* 79(2):173–180, 1998.

Soucey, M. "The Impact of Alternative Medicine and Well-Being of the Chronic Kidney Disease (CKD) Stage 5 Patient." Renal Forum. *Journal of the Americian Dietitic Association.* 27(2):1–6, Spring, 2008.

Smolinski, S. "Dietary Supplement: Adverse Reactions and Interactions. *Pharmacy Practice News.* 20–24, 1998.

Spiller, G, Spiller, M. *What's with Fiber.* Laguna Beach, CA: Basic Health Publications, 2005.

Takahashki, Y, Tanaka, A, Nakamura, T, et al. "Nicotinamide Supresses[JH1] Hypephosphatemia in Hemodialysis Patients." *Kidney International.* 65: 1099–1104, 2004.

Tyler, VE, Foster, S. "Herbs and Phytomedicinal Products[JH2]" in Covington TR(ed) *Handbook of Nonprescription Drugs,* 11th ed. American Pharmaceuticals Association, 695–713, 1996.

Walser, M, Hill, S, Tomalis, E. "Treatment of Nephrotic Adults with a Supplemented Very Low Protein Diet." *American Journal of Kidney Disease.* 28[JH3](3): 354–364, Sept 1996.

Walser, M, Mitch, W, Kopple, J, et al. "Should Protein Intake be Restricted in Pre-Dialysis Patients." *Kidney International.* 55:771–777 1999.

Wiwanitkit, V. "Renal Function Parameters of Thai Vegans Compared with Non Vegans." *Renal Failure.* 29:219–220, 2007.

Yodium, M, BenShacher, D, Ashkenazi, S, et al. "Brain iron and dopamine receptor function." In: Mandel P, De Feudis F, eds. *CNS Receptors-from Molecular Pharmacology to Behavior.* New York, NY: Raven Press, 309–321, 1983.

Young, V, Pellett, P. "Plant Proteins in Relation to Human Protein and Amino Acid Nutrition." *American Journal of Clinical Nutrition.* 59(supp):1203S–1212S, 1994.

Websites—National Institutes for Health (NIH)

http://nccam.nih.gov/health/palmetto/

http://www.nlm.nih.gov/medlineplus/druginfo/natural/patient-sawpalmetto.html

Index

Eggplant Curry, 89
Eggs, 32
Eicosapentaenoic acid (EPA),
   30, 32
Energy, 20, 64
Ensure Plus, 15
EPA. *See* Eicosapentaenoic acid
   (EPA).
Excedrin, 31
Exercise, 19, 27

F

Fajitas, 95
Fats, 6, 27–28, 42–44, 45,
   57–58
   essential, 43–44, 57
   monosaturated, 43, 44
   saturated, 42–43, 44
   trans-, 28–29, 43
Ferritin level, 20
Fiber, 6, 15, 16, 27, 28, 52, 55,
   65
Fish oil, 30, 31
Fluid intake, 14
Folic acid, 20
Foods, 16, 17, 25–26, 31, 32,
   35, 36, 38, 39, 40, 58–60
   commercial low-sodium,
   38–39
   diarrhea and, 17
   labeling of, 28, 58–59
   nausea and, 25–26
   nutrient content of, 57,
   115–117
   organic, 29
   phosphate additives in, 35
   processed, 29, 35, 37, 43, 47

processed soy-vegetarian,
   54–55
   See also Egg replacements;
   Meat replacements.
Fosrenol, 36
Fresh Corn Cakes, 94
Fruits, 16, 28, 29, 31, 40,
   55–56, 65

G

Gamma linolenic acids, 30
Garlic, 29, 65
Ginger, 67
Ginkgo, 67
Glomerular filtration rate
   (GFR), 2–3, 8, 9–11, 15,
   24, 31, 34, 61
Glomerulernephritis, 6
Glomeruli, 5
Glomerulonephritis (GN), 32
Glucerna, 15
Glucosamine sulfate, 67
Glutamine, 18
Gluten, 32, 54
Gluten-free Flour Mixture, 105
GN. *See* Glomerulonephritis
   (GN).
Grains, 7, 8, 16, 28, 56–57, 65
GRF. *See* Glomerular filtration
   rate (GFR).

H

Healing, 18–19
Heart disease, 6, 13, 20, 22,
   27–29, 35, 39, 43
Herbed Baked Eggs, 106–107

About the Author

Joan Brookhyser Hogan is a Registered Dietitian and Board-Certified Renal Nutrition Specialist. She is a frequent speaker and writer on the subject of nutrition and treatment of kidney disease, with several articles published on this subject. As a clinical dietitian for thirty years, she has extensive experience in teaching and implementing plant-based nutritional programs for those with chronic disease. She lives in Gig Harbor, Washington, with her husband, Patrick Hogan, D.O.